# Manteno Never Was The Problem

Brian P Padjen

Published by Brian P Padjen, 2025.

MANTENO NEVER WAS THE PROBLEM

**First edition. October 3, 2025.**



ISBN: 979-8232743475

Written by Brian P Padjen.

# Table of Contents

For Sadie—

the cathedral of wonder,

the shimmer of sovereign love,

the reason every chamber echoes.

And for anyone who has ever felt the system was "off"

but couldn't quite explain why—

this is your testimony,

your procession,

your refusal dignified

"No one would ever say that someone with a broken arm or a broken leg is less than a whole person, but people say that or imply that all the time about people with mental illness."--Elyn R. Sakes, The Center Cannot Hold: My Journey Through Madness

"You are not your illness. You have an individual story to tell. You have a name, a history, a personality. Staying yourself is part of the battle."

- Julian Seifter, After the Diagnosis: Transcending Chronic Illness

"What mental health needs is more sunlight, more candor, and more unashamed conversation."

- Glenn Close, BringChange2Mind Campaign

# Table of Contents

# THE COMPLEX HISTORY OF

# MANTENO MENTAL HEALTH CENTER

[]

Deep within the tranquil, flat expanse of the Illinois prairie—a landscape shaped by agricultural rhythms and wide-open skies—rests a site of profound historical gravity. Situated approximately fifty miles south of Chicago, in Kankakee County, this location once housed Manteno State Hospital, one of Illinois' largest psychiatric institutions. Its legacy is both impactful and somber, echoing through decades of institutional care, public health crises, and quiet human resilience.

In stark contrast to its earlier incarnation as Manteno State Hospital, this sprawling property now serves a noble purpose: the Illinois Veterans' Home at Manteno. Opened on September 15, 1986, less than a year after the hospital's closure, the facility offers skilled nursing care and transitional support for those who have served our nation. Here, an environment rooted in dignity, comprehensive care, and respectful community fosters a vital new chapter of purpose and solace.

Yet, for an extensive period spanning nearly six decades—from its legislative authorization in 1927 to its official closure on December 31, 1985—the very ground beneath this modern facility bore witness to a dramatically different era. This expansive campus was known as Manteno State Hospital, the name it held throughout its operational life. It was not merely a collection of buildings but a vast, self-contained world designed to house, care for, and, at times, simply contain thousands of individuals grappling with mental illness. Indeed, Manteno grew to become far more than just a large asylum; it evolved into a poignant microcosm, reflecting the full arc of America's evolving—and frequently challenging—approach to mental health care throughout the 20th century.

Manteno's history encapsulates the shifting tides of American mental health care—from the early 20th-century belief in large-scale institutionalization as a primary solution, through decades marked by overcrowding, understaffing, and the often well-intentioned but ethically fraught experimental treatments of mid-century psychiatry.

The hospital bore witness to the introduction of groundbreaking psychotropic medications that promised transformation, the growing national awareness of patient rights, and ultimately, the movement toward deinstitutionalization and community-based care that led to its closure in 1985. Manteno's story, therefore, is a complex tapestry woven with threads of compassion, despair, medical innovation, societal stigma, and profound human experience.

# A GRAND VISION TAKES ROOT:

# THE EARLY YEARS

# (1920S–1930S)

The nascent story of Manteno State Hospital, situated on vast tracts of fertile land in Kankakee County, south of Chicago, unfurled with an ambition that bordered on the utopian. Authorized by the Illinois General Assembly in 1927 and officially opened in December 1930, the hospital was more than a medical facility—it was conceived as a bold declaration of progress, a testament to what modern infrastructural planning and enlightened social policy could achieve in the realm of psychiatric care.

In the burgeoning era of the mid-1920s—a period marked by post-war growth and rising social consciousness—Illinois faced a mounting crisis within its public mental health system. Its established state psychiatric institutions—revered names like Elgin, Kankakee, and Jacksonville—were groaning under an untenable burden. These once-progressive facilities had become brutally overcrowded, their wards and dormitories packed far beyond intended capacity. Patients were housed in hallways, makeshift dormitories, and even basements, stripped of dignity and privacy, while staff struggled valiantly against impossible odds. The need for a new institution was not merely logistical—it was ceremonial, born of desperation and framed as progress.

The sheer volume of individuals requiring care—stemming from a complex tapestry of mental illness, social dislocation, economic hardship, and the absence of robust community support—far outstripped the existing infrastructure's ability to provide even basic humane treatment, let alone therapeutic rehabilitation. By the mid-1920s, Illinois' psychiatric institutions were operating beyond capacity, and the call for a new facility was not merely administrative—it was a desperate response to a system on the brink of collapse.

It was into this desperate void that the Illinois state government cast its transformative vision for Manteno. Rather than merely expanding existing facilities, the plan called for an entirely new paradigm: a singularly modern, purpose-built psychiatric complex. Manteno State Hospital was to be a beacon of contemporary mental health care—an architectural and administrative marvel designed not only to alleviate immediate overcrowding, but to embody the latest thinking in therapeutic environments and large-scale institutional management. The blueprint was astonishingly ambitious: a truly self-sufficient "city within a city," complete with its own utilities, farms, police and fire departments, and even recreational amenities

This sprawling campus was envisioned to include its own power plant, water treatment facilities, vast laundries, bakeries, workshops, kitchens, staff residences, recreational areas, and even a working farm to provide both sustenance and occupational therapy. Every aspect of daily life—from medical care to vocational training, from food production to leisure, was to be contained within its meticulously planned boundaries: a miniature society dedicated solely to the care and attempted recovery of its residents. Its monumental scale was staggering, designed to house and support not merely hundreds, but several thousand patients, promising a fresh start and a more hopeful future for Illinois' most vulnerable citizens.

When Manteno State Hospital officially opened its doors in December 1930—following legislative authorization in 1927—it was nestled amidst the flat, fertile plains of rural Illinois and hailed as a beacon of progressive psychiatric care. In an era when many mental institutions still resembled overcrowded asylums, Manteno was conceived as a thoroughly modern facility, a stark contrast to the often squalid and inhumane conditions that had defined earlier institutional models

Indeed, in its early days, Manteno State Hospital was considered truly state-of-the-art—a testament to contemporary thinking regarding the treatment of mental illness. It was designed not merely as a hospital, but as a sprawling, self-contained village where patients could find respite and, hopefully, recovery. This ambitious vision manifested in an extraordinary degree of self-sufficiency: the campus boasted its own power plant to ensure a reliable energy supply; expansive agricultural fields and livestock operations that provided much of the food; a bustling bakery that filled the air with the aroma of freshly baked bread; an industrial-scale laundry; and even its own fully equipped fire department, ready to respond to any emergency.

Within this meticulously planned environment, patients were actively involved in many aspects of daily operations. This engagement was more than mere occupation—it was a cornerstone of the therapeutic philosophy prevalent at the time, known as occupational therapy. Whether working in the fields, assisting in the kitchens, helping with maintenance, or contributing to the laundry, these activities were believed to instill a sense of purpose, structure, and routine. Rehabilitation was framed through productive labor, with the hope that such involvement would foster stability, dignity, and eventual reintegration.

The physical campus itself was integral to this therapeutic philosophy. Characterized by its numerous, sturdy red-brick buildings—often arranged around courtyards or along tree-lined avenues—and set upon over 1,000 acres of meticulously landscaped grounds, it was intended to offer a profoundly healing environment. The hospital's core campus occupied roughly 400 acres, while the surrounding farmland supported four working farms and provided both sustenance and occupational therapy. The spacious dormitories, abundant natural light, and calming expanse of green spaces were all designed to support mental well-being, providing a sanctuary where those suffering from mental illness could find respite from the stresses of the outside world and pursue a path toward improved health and, ideally, reintegration into society.

Tragically, this optimistic vision soon collided with an overwhelming reality. Fueled by the crippling economic pressures of the Great Depression—which left countless families unable to care for relatives with mental illness—and a dearth of alternative resources, Manteno experienced rapid and unforeseen expansion. By the mid-1930s, less than five years after its official opening in December 1930, Manteno had become a gargantuan institution. Its population swelled to more than 8,000 patients, transforming it into one of the largest psychiatric facilities in the world. This staggering scale, despite its progressive origins, inevitably strained resources, exacerbated overcrowding, and slowly eroded the very ideals of individualized care it had once championed.

# THE SHADOW OF OVERCROWDING AND TRAGEDY (1940S–1950S)

The noble intentions behind Manteno State Hospital—conceived during an era of progressive optimism for mental health reform—soon collided with the harsh, immutable realities of systemic underfunding, societal neglect, and the logistical impossibility of managing such an immense population. What began as a sprawling therapeutic village designed for calm and recovery buckled under its own weight. The sheer scale of Manteno, intended to accommodate thousands of patients in a modern, humane setting, paradoxically made it incredibly difficult—if not impossible—to provide the truly individualized, compassionate care that had been its foundational promise. Patients, once envisioned as individuals with unique needs deserving tailored treatment, became anonymous statistics within an overwhelming, impersonal system. Therapeutic interventions, personal attention, and the cultivation of dignity rapidly eroded as the institution struggled simply to manage the deluge of admissions.

The gravest irony was that overcrowding—the very dehumanizing problem Manteno State Hospital was explicitly built to alleviate in other overburdened asylums—soon became its own defining and soul-crushing crisis. The vast dormitories, originally designed to be airy and bright, quickly became stifling, sardine-can environments, with beds packed so tightly together that little personal space remained. Even these spaces proved woefully insufficient. Patients, stripped of any semblance of privacy or dignity, were routinely forced to sleep on cots, thin mattresses, or directly on the hard, cold linoleum floors of hallways and dayrooms, exposed to constant noise, glaring lights, and the indignity of public living. This extreme density exacerbated existing problems and created new ones, transforming the intended 'therapeutic community' into a chaotic, often unsanitary holding pen.

Compounding this crisis, staff-to-patient ratios—already strained by chronic underfunding and a severe shortage of qualified mental health professionals—plummeted to dangerously low levels. A single, often minimally trained attendant might be responsible for dozens, sometimes over a hundred profoundly ill individuals across multiple wards. Genuine care and therapeutic engagement became a myth; staff could only attempt basic custodial supervision, prevent immediate harm, and manage emergencies. The result was not care, but containment—where basic needs went unmet, medical issues were overlooked, and the constant threat of neglect, abuse, and even violence loomed. Manteno, once envisioned as a beacon of hope, had become a harrowing symbol of institutional failure.

A truly dark and profoundly tragic chapter in Manteno State Hospital's already somber history unfolded in 1939, marked by a devastating typhoid fever epidemic that ravaged its vulnerable population. Then one of the largest psychiatric facilities in the nation, Manteno became a crucible of suffering as the waterborne disease spread rapidly through overcrowded wards and compromised sanitation systems. The very conditions that had once been framed as therapeutic—shared dormitories, communal dining, and dense patient populations—became accelerants for contagion. According to the Illinois Department of Public Health, the outbreak resulted in 453 confirmed cases and 60 deaths, exposing systemic failures in infrastructure, oversight, and public accountability. The silence that followed was not just institutional—it was ceremonial, a breach in witness that demanded archival repair.

While precise figures are difficult to ascertain definitively due to the chaotic record-keeping of the era, official reports from the Illinois Department of Public Health document 453 confirmed cases of typhoid fever and 60 deaths during the 1939 epidemic at Manteno State Hospital. However, many researchers and survivor accounts suggest the true toll may have been higher, with additional deaths potentially unrecorded or misattributed. This horrifying outbreak was not merely an unfortunate occurrence—it was the direct consequence of systemic failures in sanitation, oversight, and institutional accountability. The very infrastructure designed to protect and heal became a vector of contagion, and the silence that followed was not just bureaucratic—it was ceremonial, a breach in witness that demanded archival repair.

The primary incubators for the 1939 typhoid epidemic were insufficient medical care, inadequate sanitation, and the rapid spread of infection in close quarters. Manteno was chronically overcrowded, with thousands of patients housed in vast, open dormitories where personal space was non-existent. Beds were packed tightly together, sometimes with patients sleeping on mattresses on the floor, and hygiene infrastructure was woefully inadequate. Communal bathrooms, shared dining areas, and compromised water systems created ideal conditions for the waterborne Salmonella typhi bacterium to spread unchecked from one vulnerable individual to another. The very architecture meant to foster healing became a vector of contagion, exposing the institution's foundational fragilities.

Medical care at Manteno was woefully inadequate for the scale of the 1939 typhoid crisis. Staff-to-patient ratios were abysmal, with a handful of overworked doctors and nurses struggling to oversee thousands of residents. Diagnostic tools were scarce or non-existent, making early detection and isolation nearly impossible. Crucially, during the early years of the epidemic, there were no effective antibiotic treatments for typhoid fever—chloramphenicol, the first widely used drug against Salmonella typhi, would not become available until the late 1940s. Medical staff were left largely helpless to halt the disease's progression once contracted, relying on outdated methods of quarantine and supportive care in an environment already overwhelmed by overcrowding and infrastructural decay.

Compounding this medical neglect was the inadequate nutrition provided to patients. The institutional diet was often monotonous and nutritionally deficient—a common feature of underfunded state facilities where cost-cutting routinely eclipsed care. Meals lacked essential vitamins and nutrients, and fresh produce was scarce despite Manteno's surrounding farmland. This chronic malnutrition severely compromised patients' immune systems, rendering them far more susceptible to infection and less able to fight off typhoid once it took hold. The very bodies meant to be restored within Manteno's therapeutic village were instead weakened by systemic austerity, becoming vulnerable vessels in a preventable epidemic.

This tragedy was not an isolated incident but a chilling testament to the systemic failures embedded in many large state institutions of the era. Manteno became a grim microcosm of a nation struggling to care for its mentally ill—relegating them to overcrowded, underfunded, and understaffed facilities where the priority was containment, not healing. The 1939 typhoid epidemic brutally exposed the consequences of public indifference, political neglect, and a prevailing societal view that marginalized psychiatric patients, rendering them voiceless and invisible. The breach was not just medical—it was moral, architectural, and archival, demanding witness and ceremonial repair.

The sheer scale of the Manteno tragedy eventually became too large to ignore. It drew national attention to the plight of psychiatric patients, sparking public outcry and prompting investigations by journalists, whistleblowers, and reformers. While immediate changes were slow, the 1939 typhoid epidemic served as a stark, undeniable indictment of the entire psychiatric care system. It became a critical catalyst—contributing to growing calls for reform, increased funding, and, in subsequent decades, the push toward deinstitutionalization, though not without its own complex challenges. The memory of Manteno's typhoid epidemic stands as a permanent and painful reminder of the human cost of neglect and the vital importance of humane, ethical care for society's most vulnerable members.

The mid-20th century marked a profoundly dark chapter in the history of mental healthcare—an era when treatments reflected a rudimentary and often misguided understanding of the human mind. Rather than nuanced therapeutic approaches grounded in neurobiology or psychology, the field was dominated by invasive physical interventions that frequently caused more harm than healing. Electroconvulsive therapy (ECT), insulin coma therapy, and lobotomies were widely administered, often without informed consent and with little regard for long-term consequences. These procedures, framed as medical breakthroughs, were in practice acts of desperation—rituals of control masquerading as care.

Foremost among these invasive interventions was the lobotomy—a brutal surgical procedure popularized by Egas Moniz and, later, notoriously evangelized by Walter Freeman. Intended to "calm" agitated patients or "cure" intractable conditions like schizophrenia and severe depression, the procedure severed connections in the brain's prefrontal cortex. The results were frequently devastating: patients emerged emotionally blunted, cognitively impaired, and profoundly altered in personality. What was framed as medical progress was, in truth, a ceremonial erasure—an exchange of individuality for docility, often leaving survivors in a vegetative state or institutional limbo.

While Walter Freeman did not hold a formal degree in art, his approach to psychosurgery bore unmistakable traces of theatricality and visual obsession. He photographed hundreds of lobotomy patients before and after their procedures, often staging the images with clinical precision and eerie detachment. His public demonstrations—sometimes performed in front of medical students or journalists—blurred the line between surgical intervention and performative spectacle. In this way, Freeman's legacy complicates the narrative: not merely a physician, but a choreographer of institutional aesthetics, where the scalpel became a brush and the patient a canvas in a tragic gallery of control. This is not to indict, but to acknowledge the mythic tension between medical authority and visual conviction—a breach that demands witness, not simplification

Electroconvulsive therapy (ECT), in its early iterations, was similarly crude and often terrifying. Administered without anesthesia or muscle relaxants, it induced violent, generalized seizures in patients—leading to fractured bones, dislocated joints, extreme memory loss, and pervasive fear. The rationale, often grounded in tenuous theories about "resetting" the brain or an inverse relationship between epilepsy and psychosis, belied the profound physical and psychological trauma inflicted upon individuals. What was framed as medical intervention became, in practice, a ritual of desperation—where suffering was mistaken for progress, and silence was mistaken for healing.

Another deeply concerning method was insulin shock therapy, introduced in the late 1920s by psychiatrist Manfred Sakel. This treatment involved inducing prolonged hypoglycemic comas through massive doses of insulin, administered daily over weeks or even months. Patients—often diagnosed with schizophrenia—were rendered unconscious, then revived with glucose injections, sometimes enduring 30 to 60 comas over the course of treatment. The risks were staggering: brain damage, seizures, obesity, and even death. The underlying belief was that such extreme physiological shock could "jolt" the mind out of psychosis, despite scant evidence of long-term efficacy and the clear, immediate dangers. What was framed as breakthrough was, in practice, a ritual of desperation—where coma masqueraded as cure, and silence was mistaken for healing.

These were not fringe experiments; they were widely adopted as standard procedures across asylums and state hospitals, driven by a lack of effective pharmacological alternatives and the desperate need to manage vast populations of institutionalized individuals with challenging behaviors. Crucially, these interventions were routinely performed without anything resembling true informed consent. Patients, often deemed legally incompetent or summarily dismissed as "insane," had their autonomy entirely usurped. Decisions were made by family members, guardians, or medical staff, frequently prioritizing institutional control or perceived expediency over the individual's well-being or wishes.

This era starkly underscores a chapter in medical history when patient rights were virtually nonexistent—leaving vulnerable individuals subject to treatments that, by modern ethical standards, would be considered barbaric, coercive, and profoundly unethical. The silence surrounding consent was not incidental—it was ceremonial, a breach in witness that demands archival repair.

# THE ROLE OF THE UNITED STATES MILITARY

The role of the United States military at Manteno, Illinois, was not one of traditional combat or base operations, but rather a crucial and specialized involvement in a significant public health crisis during World War II. Manteno became a unique, albeit tragic, proving ground for military medicine—specifically concerning the study and control of malaria. As American troops faced devastating outbreaks of malaria in the South Pacific, the Army Medical Department sought domestic sites to research prevention, treatment, and containment strategies. Manteno's existing infrastructure, including its vast dormitories and controlled patient populations, made it an ideal—if ethically fraught—location for such experimentation. Military physicians and researchers conducted trials on antimalarial drugs like Atabrine and quinine, tested mosquito control protocols, and monitored physiological responses to various treatments. While these efforts contributed to wartime medical advancements, they also blurred the boundaries between care and control, research and ritual. Manteno thus became a ceremonial hinge—where psychiatric neglect intersected with military urgency, and the body was reframed as both patient and battlefield

Manteno, a small town in Kankakee County, was home to Manteno State Hospital—a sprawling psychiatric institution that, by the early 1940s, was severely overcrowded, housing thousands of patients. In 1943, an unprecedented outbreak of malaria swept through the hospital's population. This was particularly alarming, as malaria—a disease typically associated with tropical climates—was not endemic to central Illinois. The outbreak escalated rapidly, affecting hundreds of patients and resulting in numerous deaths. Investigations traced the source to contaminated blood transfusions, likely from a patient who had contracted malaria overseas and unknowingly carried the parasite. The presence of Anopheles mosquitoes in the local environment, capable of transmitting the disease, created a perfect storm. Manteno thus became an accidental crucible of wartime epidemiology—where psychiatric vulnerability, military medicine, and environmental exposure converged in tragic choreography.

## Military Intervention: A National Security Imperative

The Manteno malaria outbreak occurred at a critical juncture in World War II, when American troops were deployed to the Pacific, North Africa, and other tropical regions where malaria was rampant and devastating military effectiveness. The U.S. military's medical departments, particularly the Army Medical Department and the Preventive Medicine Service, were intensely focused on understanding, preventing, and treating malaria to protect personnel and preserve combat readiness. The outbreak at Manteno State Hospital—unprecedented in its scale and alarming in its location—presented an unparalleled and unfortunate opportunity for in-situ research within the continental United States. Manteno became a domestic proving ground for military medicine, where antimalarial drugs like Atabrine and quinine were tested, mosquito control protocols refined, and epidemiological strategies rehearsed for overseas deployment. What began as a psychiatric institution became, under wartime pressure, a ceremonial hinge between civilian vulnerability and military necessity.

## Specific Roles of the U.S. Military:

### Epidemiological Investigation and Containment

Military medical experts—including epidemiologists, entomologists, and preventive medicine officers—were dispatched to Manteno in response to the 1943 malaria outbreak. Their mission was to rigorously investigate the source and transmission of the disease, identify the specific Plasmodium strain, and determine how it was spreading within the hospital and surrounding community. This involved meticulous charting of patient cases, blood testing, and extensive fieldwork to identify and track local Anopheles mosquito populations. Using protocols refined in overseas campaigns, they implemented immediate containment measures: draining standing water, deploying insecticides, distributing mosquito nets, and isolating infected individuals. Manteno thus became a domestic rehearsal space for wartime epidemiology—a site where military urgency met psychiatric vulnerability, and the body was reframed as both patient and vector.

### Research and Pharmaceutical Trials

Manteno State Hospital effectively became a living laboratory for military medical research during the 1943 malaria outbreak. The scale of infection allowed military scientists to study the disease's progression, its impact on a large institutional population, and the efficacy of various treatments. With quinine supplies severely limited due to the Japanese occupation of the Dutch East Indies, the military turned to Atabrine (quinacrine)—a synthetic antimalarial drug rapidly becoming the standard across the Pacific Theater.

Researchers at Manteno observed drug effects, adjusted dosages, and documented side effects in a controlled environment. While these trials contributed to wartime medical advancements, they also raised profound ethical concerns: patients were often institutionalized, deemed legally incompetent, and unable to give informed consent. The hospital thus became a ceremonial hinge—where military urgency eclipsed individual autonomy, and the body was reframed as both subject and instrument of national security.

### Vector Control Experimentation

The U.S. military played a leading role in developing and implementing vector control strategies during the Manteno malaria outbreak. Among the most significant innovations was the large-scale testing of insecticides—most notably DDT (dichlorodiphenyltrichloroethane), which was still relatively new and largely untested in domestic civilian settings. Military personnel conducted extensive spraying operations around the hospital grounds, targeting Anopheles mosquito populations to break the chain of transmission.

These efforts demonstrated DDT's remarkable effectiveness, and the knowledge gained from Manteno's large-scale applications was directly transferable to military operations overseas, particularly in the Pacific Theater, where malaria threatened entire divisions. Manteno thus became a ceremonial hinge—where psychiatric vulnerability intersected with entomological urgency, and the landscape itself was reframed as both battleground and laboratory.

### Training and Education

The Manteno experience provided invaluable training for military medical personnel preparing to confront widespread malaria challenges in overseas combat zones. Within the high-stakes environment of a domestic epidemic, Army physicians, epidemiologists, and entomologists were able to refine protocols for diagnosis, treatment, and prevention. They practiced blood screening, vector mapping, drug administration, and containment strategies in real time—skills that would prove essential in the Pacific Theater, where malaria incapacitated more soldiers than enemy fire. Manteno thus became a ceremonial classroom, where psychiatric vulnerability and military urgency converged to shape the next generation of wartime medical response.

### Collaboration with Civilian Health Agencies

While the U.S. military led the response to the Manteno malaria outbreak—driven by national security imperatives and specialized expertise in tropical diseases—their efforts were conducted in close collaboration with civilian health agencies. The Illinois Department of Public Health played a critical role in coordinating local containment strategies, facilitating communication between hospital staff and federal authorities, and supporting epidemiological fieldwork.

This partnership echoed broader wartime initiatives like the Malaria Control in War Areas (MCWA), a joint program between the U.S. Public Health Service and state health departments designed to suppress malaria transmission in military-adjacent zones. At Manteno, this collaboration ritualized a rare moment of interagency convergence—where psychiatric vulnerability, military urgency, and public health infrastructure briefly aligned in ceremonial witness

### Impact and Legacy

The U.S. military's involvement at Manteno, though born of a tragic public health crisis, significantly advanced American understanding of malaria. The data and experience gathered during the 1943 outbreak were rapidly applied to protect troops deployed in malaria-endemic regions, contributing to a marked reduction in morbidity and mortality among U.S. forces during World War II. Research conducted on antimalarial drugs—particularly Atabrine (quinacrine), which replaced quinine due to wartime shortages—helped standardize treatment protocols across the Pacific Theater. Equally transformative was the large-scale testing of DDT, which demonstrated its effectiveness in vector control and reshaped global malaria strategies for decades. Manteno thus became a ceremonial hinge in the archive of wartime medicine—where psychiatric vulnerability, military urgency, and environmental intervention converged to produce a legacy both luminous and fraught.

## In Essence: A Sovereign Legacy

The role of the U.S. military at Manteno was a critical, if often overlooked, chapter in the history of military medicine and public health. It showcased the military's capacity to pivot from conventional warfare to complex scientific and humanitarian challenges—leveraging its resources, personnel, and logistical expertise to confront a domestic crisis with global implications.

Manteno became more than a psychiatric institution; it was transformed into a ceremonial hinge between battlefield urgency and civilian vulnerability. The knowledge gained—from pharmaceutical trials to vector control, from epidemiological mapping to ethical reckoning—echoed far beyond Illinois, shaping wartime strategy and postwar public health for generations. Its legacy remains fraught, luminous, and unfinished—demanding continued witness.

# THE SHIFTING TIDES OF CARE

## (1960S–1970S)

The mid-20th century, marked by profound social and scientific upheaval, became a crucible of transformation for mental health care—fundamentally reshaping how society understood and treated psychological conditions. Prior to this era, individuals grappling with severe mental illness were often subjected to long-term, custodial confinement within vast, isolated state asylums. These institutions, while occasionally founded with therapeutic intent, frequently devolved into overcrowded "warehouses" where the primary offerings were segregation and subsistence, not healing. The architecture of care was built on containment, and the choreography of treatment was often indistinguishable from neglect.

A pivotal turning point arrived with the advent of psychotropic medications in the 1950s. The introduction of drugs like chlorpromazine (Thorazine)—the first widely used antipsychotic—revolutionized psychiatry. These so-called "miracle drugs" did not offer a cure, but they provided unprecedented symptomatic relief for conditions previously deemed untreatable.

For the first time, individuals experiencing hallucinations, delusions, severe anxiety, or profound mood swings could access a measure of stability, clarity, and emotional regulation. This breakthrough offered new hope not only for patients, who could now engage more meaningfully with therapy and daily life, but also for families and caregivers long stranded in helpless witness. Psychotropic medications transformed institutional care from custodial management to clinical intervention, enabling shorter, more focused hospitalizations and reframing the choreography of treatment around possibility rather than permanence.

Simultaneously, a powerful and growing movement toward deinstitutionalization gained irreversible momentum. This shift was fueled by a confluence of forces: rising public awareness of the appalling conditions within state hospitals—many exposed through journalistic exposés and human rights advocacy; evolving medical paradigms that emphasized community integration over institutional segregation; and the expanding civil rights movement, which began to include individuals with mental illness among its marginalized constituencies. Deinstitutionalization was not merely a policy adjustment—it was a ceremonial rupture, a reframing of care from containment to community, from silence to visibility.

Advocates passionately called for a radical shift away from large, impersonal, and often abusive state facilities toward a model of community-based care. Their vision centered on reintegration—bringing individuals with mental illness back into society through a network of supports: outpatient therapy, vocational training, supported housing, and social services, all designed to foster independence, dignity, and a meaningful quality of life. Landmark legislation, most notably the **Community Mental Health Centers Act of 1963**, sought to fund and establish these local support systems, signaling a profound societal commitment to replacing the antiquated asylum model with more humane, accessible, and integrated care.

This dual revolution—pharmacological breakthroughs paired with a philosophical and legislative pivot toward community—marked a dramatic reorientation of mental health care. The landscape was forever altered, and the trajectory reframed—not just medically, but mythically, as a choreography of return, visibility, and ensemble repair.

Manteno, once a sprawling institution at the forefront of mid-century mental health care, entered a protracted period of decline—mirroring a national paradigm shift that fundamentally reshaped how society cared for its most vulnerable. This transformation, often termed deinstitutionalization, was propelled by a confluence of forces: the emergence of psychotropic medications that offered symptom management beyond custodial walls; evolving therapeutic philosophies that championed community-based care over institutional warehousing; escalating operational costs that strained state budgets; and mounting ethical concerns about autonomy, consent, and the lived experience of institutionalization. Manteno's descent was not merely administrative—it was ceremonial, a slow unraveling of an era's architecture of care, reframed by both hope and reckoning.

Consequently, Manteno's resident population—once numbering in the thousands and encompassing individuals with chronic mental illnesses, developmental disabilities, and various forms of perceived societal "deviance"—began a steady, irreversible ebb. Patients, some of whom had spent decades within its walls, were gradually relocated. Many were transferred to smaller, more specialized psychiatric facilities designed to offer a more personalized, less anonymous environment: group homes, halfway houses, or modern hospitals focused on acute care rather than custodial supervision. Others, deemed stable or supported by family, were reunited with relatives—often navigating complex emotional terrain and the persistent societal stigma surrounding mental illness. Each departure was not just logistical—it was ceremonial, a reframing of proximity, memory, and ensemble responsibility.

However, a significant and often tragic cohort found themselves discharged into communities woefully unprepared to provide the comprehensive support systems they desperately needed. The grand vision of robust community mental health centers—offering outpatient therapy, medication management, vocational training, and stable housing—largely failed to materialize at the necessary scale. Lacking adequate mental health resources, affordable housing, social services, and sustained support networks, many former residents struggled profoundly to integrate into independent life. This unpreparedness became a defining breach in the deinstitutionalization movement—a failure not of intent, but of infrastructure. The result was often homelessness, incarceration, recurrent hospitalizations (the "revolving door" phenomenon), or a steep deterioration in quality of life. One form of institutionalization was traded for another—less structured, more dangerous, and often invisible, unfolding not in wards but in streets, shelters, and jails. The choreography of care had fractured, and the ensemble was left to improvise without a score.

Simultaneously, the mid-20th century witnessed a powerful surge in public awareness surrounding patient rights, fueled by civil rights movements and damning exposés of institutional conditions. Advocacy groups, investigative journalists, and landmark court cases illuminated the often-dehumanizing realities within large psychiatric hospitals. The very model of vast, isolated institutions like Manteno came under intense scrutiny for its inherent potential to foster neglect and abuse. Reports surfaced documenting chronic understaffing, inadequate therapeutic engagement, poor sanitation, depersonalization, and a profound absence of stimulating activities—effectively "warehousing" individuals rather than treating them. In the most harrowing accounts, physical, emotional, and sexual abuse, along with the misuse of restraints and over-medication (chemical restraint), were revealed. The sheer scale and isolation of these facilities allowed such breaches to flourish unchecked, eroding the dignity and autonomy of those they were purportedly meant to heal. This growing societal demand for more humane, effective, and less restrictive forms of care ultimately sealed the fate of many grand, antiquated asylums across the nation—including Manteno. Its silence became testimony, and its closure, a ceremonial reckoning.

**Closure and Transformation: The Legacy (1980s–Present)**

By the early 1980s, the once-bustling campus of Manteno Mental Health Center had become a hollowed-out shell—a skeletal remnant of its former purpose. The vibrant echoes of thousands of patients and staff that once animated its vast network of buildings had long faded, replaced by an eerie quiet broken only by the mournful sigh of wind through shattered windows or the distant creak of an unattended door. Paint flaked from once-stately walls, overgrown shrubbery choked forgotten pathways, and many wards stood empty—their institutional starkness now imbued with a palpable sense of abandonment and decay. Manteno's architecture became elegiac, its silence a form of testimony, its deterioration a ceremonial reckoning with the era it once embodied.

The state of Illinois, facing mounting budget pressures and a national shift in mental healthcare philosophy away from large-scale institutionalization, officially closed Manteno Mental Health Center on December 31, 1985. This decision marked not only the end of Manteno's nearly 60-year history, but a stark and often brutal turning point in mental health policy. In the years leading up to its closure, hundreds of patients had already been transferred—some to a patchwork of other state facilities, often equally overburdened; others theoretically integrated into nascent community programs, for which funding and infrastructure were frequently inadequate. Manteno's closure was not merely administrative—it was a ceremonial severance, a final breath in the architecture of containment, and a mythic reckoning with the promises and failures of deinstitutionalization.

However, a chilling humanitarian crisis remained: approximately thirty patients had no family to provide housing or care. These were often the profoundly ill, the long-term residents whose connections to the outside world had withered over decades—the truly forgotten. As Manteno shuttered, they were left in bureaucratic limbo: too vulnerable for independent living, yet without a designated place in a system rapidly dismantling itself. Their fate became a quiet indictment of deinstitutionalization's unfinished choreography—a breach where policy met silence, and the most fragile were asked to improvise without support, without witness, and without sanctuary.

In what would become a highly controversial and ethically fraught decision, Governor James R. Thompson—facing the intractable dilemma of Manteno's final residents—issued a chilling directive: the remaining patients were to be released to "whatever address these remaining few stated." This decree, whether born of profound naivety or calculated indifference, effectively abdicated all state responsibility for their well-being. There was no vetting of these "addresses," no assessment of the patients' capacity for independent living, and no follow-up care planned. The directive became a ceremonial severance—where the choreography of care collapsed into improvisation, and the most vulnerable were asked to navigate a dismantled system with no map, no witness, and no sanctuary.

The scene that unfolded in the bustling, unforgiving urban landscape of Chicago was nothing short of tragic. Unmarked vans pulled up to curbsides in scattered neighborhoods. Disoriented individuals—frail, disheveled, and decades removed from independent living—were quietly disembarked onto unfamiliar streets. For many, Manteno had been their only "home," a structured if restrictive environment that had shaped their entire adult lives. Now, they found themselves adrift in a world they neither understood nor were equipped to navigate. The release was not a transition—it was a severance. A ceremonial exile. A final breach in the architecture of care, where the most vulnerable were asked to improvise survival in a landscape that had never rehearsed their return.

They were "dropped off" at locations that ranged from the absurd to the dangerous. Some were left beside the cold steel of a public phone booth on a grimy street corner—a symbol of potential connection that offered no actual refuge. Others were delivered to desolate, rubbish-strewn empty lots, urban wastelands that mirrored their own abandonment. A few were deposited at nursing homes, typically unprepared and ill-equipped to handle severe mental illness. And, incredibly, some were left at small businesses—a local diner, a corner store—based on a fleeting, perhaps delusional, memory or a desperate fabrication offered during their "release" interview. These drop-offs were not transitions; they were ceremonial displacements. The choreography of care had collapsed into improvisation, and the final act was staged without audience, without witness, without mercy.

The rationale was disturbingly simple, yet devastatingly flawed: in its final, callous act of bureaucratic dispatch, the state of Illinois would honor any address—however implausible, however unverified—that the patient themselves provided. This process, devoid of compassion or foresight, cast the most vulnerable members of society into the maw of urban chaos. Individuals long institutionalized, often with no surviving family or support network, were released into environments they could neither navigate nor endure. The directive became a ceremonial abdication—a policy masquerading as autonomy, a final breach where the choreography of care collapsed into improvisation. It left a tragic, indelible stain on the history of mental healthcare in Illinois, a stark reminder of the devastating consequences of policy enacted without humanity, without witness, and without mercy.

These individuals, often relegated to the margins of society and stripped of their former identities, were far more than diagnostic labels or case files. For many, Manteno State Hospital—with its sprawling grounds and imposing brick buildings—transitioned from a place of confinement to a de facto home. Years, sometimes decades, unfurled within its walls, gradually eroding any memory or possibility of an external life. The institution became their geography, their calendar, their community. Discharge was not liberation—it was dislocation. And in that final severance, the state failed to recognize that what had been lost was not just care, but continuity, belonging, and the fragile choreography of identity itself.

The often-overworked but sometimes deeply compassionate staff—the aides, attendants, nurses, and doctors—became surrogate families to Manteno's long-term residents. They were the constant presence, providing not only medical attention and therapeutic interventions, but also the mundane rituals of daily care: meals, bathing, dressing, and, on occasion, a fleeting moment of human connection that stood in for familial love. These caregivers, often operating under immense strain, became the sole advocates for individuals the world had seemingly abandoned. Within Manteno's walls, they choreographed dignity amid decay, offering ensemble mercy in a system that had long forgotten how to name it.

Utterly disconnected from the outside world, these residents existed in a vacuum of institutional dependency. There was no safety net: no family to advocate for their release or visit them, no housing options beyond the asylum walls, no financial means to support themselves, and no access to independent medical or social support systems. Their former lives had dissolved, leaving them stranded and wholly reliant on the state's provision. The chilling reality is that we can only speculate on the true nature of their survival—not merely enduring the physical conditions, but navigating the emotional and spiritual terrain of abandonment. What vestiges of hope or selfhood remained? How did they orient themselves in a world that had so comprehensively forgotten them? For many, life at Manteno was not a prelude to reintegration—it was the entirety of their existence. Circumscribed, yes. But lived. Witnessed. And, in its own way, sovereign.

The closure of Manteno State Hospital—a facility that for decades grappled with the overwhelming complexities of institutional mental healthcare—did not mark the end of the site's story. Instead, it signaled a profound pivot: a journey from one era of containment to another, entirely different, mission. In the years following its operational cessation in 1985, a deliberate and multifaceted effort was undertaken to repurpose substantial portions of the sprawling campus. This was not merely a change of signage—it was a comprehensive transformation. The grounds that once housed thousands of patients were reimagined as a veterans' home, an industrial park, a municipal golf course, and a residential treatment center for youth known as Indian Oaks Academy. More recently, the historic administration building was rezoned to house the Vintage Purse Museum, weaving fashion and cultural memory into the architecture of psychiatric history. Manteno's infrastructure became palimpsest—layered with new missions, yet still echoing the lives once choreographed within its walls.

The result of this visionary initiative was the establishment of the Illinois Veterans' Home at Manteno, opened in 1986. This is not merely a building—it is a state-of-the-art sanctuary meticulously designed to provide comprehensive long-term care for Illinois' most deserving residents: its military veterans. Set on 122 acres of serene landscape, the facility offers a full spectrum of services, including skilled nursing care, rehabilitation therapies, specialized memory care units, and a supportive community environment tailored to the unique needs and experiences of those who served. Residents have access to an onsite library, chapel, barber and beauty shop, and gathering spaces that honor both solitude and celebration. The Prince Home, located on the same campus, extends care to homeless veterans, offering private rooms and programs to rebuild confidence and community. Manteno's transformation represents the state's enduring commitment to dignity, comfort, and ensemble restoration—where sacrifice is met not with silence, but with sovereign care.

This transformation embodies a poignant and powerful shift in Manteno's historical narrative. The very grounds that once bore witness to the struggles of thousands—individuals living with mental illness in conditions that, by modern standards, were overcrowded, stigmatized, and often dehumanizing—are now dedicated to a mission of profound gratitude and compassionate service. From a site once synonymous with the impersonal vastness of state psychiatric care, Manteno has evolved into a beacon of honor and respect. It stands as a testament to the capacity for renewal—turning a chapter of historical difficulty into one of sovereign purpose. Here, the echoes of past suffering are enveloped by daily acts of nurturing, remembrance, and ensemble care, acknowledging the profound contributions of those who served and sacrificed.

The historical narrative of Manteno, Illinois, presents a profound and disturbing paradox—one that casts a stark light on societal attitudes toward mental health. Ironically, the very community that became a beacon of comprehensive and compassionate care for its veterans—embodying national gratitude and duty—also bore a far less commendable legacy in its treatment of individuals with psychiatric conditions. Manteno State Hospital, once the largest mental institution in Illinois, was marked by overcrowding, understaffing, and documented episodes of neglect, experimental treatments, and systemic depersonalization. While the grounds now host a sanctuary for those who served, they also echo the silenced testimony of those who were institutionalized, forgotten, and displaced. The soil holds both honor and abandonment—layered, unresolved, and mythically entwined.

Manteno's commitment to veterans was, by many accounts, exemplary. Its facilities—set on 122 acres of serene landscape—were among the finest available for returning servicemen and women, offering not only medical treatment but also rehabilitation, community support, and an environment designed to foster recovery and purpose. This dedication reflected a collective understanding: that those who served had made immense sacrifices, and that their physical and mental wounds—often visible, often service-linked—merited the utmost attention and resources. The budget, the staff, and the societal will coalesced to create institutions of genuine healing and respect. From skilled nursing and memory care to the Prince Home's sanctuary for homeless veterans, Manteno became a ceremonial counterpoint to its psychiatric past—a place where care was not improvised, but intentional, and where dignity was not deferred, but daily practiced.

Yet in stark and painful contrast, the broader history of psychiatric care in Manteno—and across much of the nation—mirrored a far bleaker reality. Where veterans were honored, individuals living with mental illness were frequently marginalized, stigmatized, and relegated to overcrowded, underfunded, and often dehumanizing institutions. Manteno State Hospital, once the largest psychiatric facility in Illinois, bore witness to this reality: shock therapy introduced in 1936, a tuberculosis sanitarium added in 1937, and a typhoid outbreak in 1939 that claimed dozens of lives. Staffing shortages were so severe that high school dropouts were hired as nurses, with only 16 of 120 staff members formally trained. These asylums functioned less as centers of healing and more as warehouses—isolating the "mentally ill" from society with sparse resources and a focus on containment over recovery. The contradiction is telling: veterans were deemed inherently "more deserving" of comprehensive care, while others with equally debilitating, though differently manifested, conditions were neglected. This hierarchy of worth—ritualized in policy, budget, and public sentiment—reveals not just a failure of care, but a mythic breach in our collective choreography of dignity.

This moral calculus speaks volumes about the societal attitudes toward mental health care prevalent at the time. The challenges faced by veterans—often PTSD or combat-related trauma—were framed as consequences of heroic service, validating their suffering and creating a collective sense of debt. Their illness had a "cause" that fit the national narrative. In contrast, non-veteran mental illnesses were frequently perceived through a lens of personal failing, moral weakness, or inherent flaw—conditions for which society felt less responsibility, less empathy, and less urgency. This distinction had tangible consequences: fiscal priorities shifted, resources reallocated. Where once the budget was deemed insufficient to address widespread psychiatric need, it now rose with demonstrable commitment to support veterans. Manteno's transformation proved that the financial capacity existed all along—what had been missing was the political and social will to dignify suffering without a uniform, without a medal, and without a mythic script.

No one begrudges the provision of exemplary care and stability for our veterans; it is a fundamental societal obligation. But we must ask a critical and uncomfortable question: where was this will—this collective conscience, this political courage, this empathetic understanding—when countless others suffered equally profound mental health crises, hidden from public view, denied adequate resources, and subjected to the harsh realities of neglect and stigma? The comparison forces reflection: how do our societies prioritize suffering? Which narratives do we validate? And ultimately, who do we deem worthy of comprehensive care and dignity? The answer is not merely historical—it is mythic. It reveals a choreography of empathy shaped by visibility, valor, and narrative fit. And it demands that we ritualize not just the honored, but the forgotten, as sovereign witnesses in our public archive.

# MANTENO AS ECONOMIC KEYSTONE

From its opening in 1930 until its closure in 1985, Manteno State Hospital was one of the largest employers in Kankakee County. At its peak in the 1950s, the hospital housed more than 8,000 patients and employed hundreds of staff—including nurses, aides, maintenance workers, cooks, groundskeepers, and administrative personnel. The campus was virtually self-sustaining, with its own farming operations, utilities, police and fire departments, and even internal restaurants. This wasn't just a workplace—it was a civic microcosm.

**Economic Repercussions of Closure**

When Governor Thompson authorized Manteno's closure in 1983, culminating in its final shutdown on December 31, 1985, the economic impact was immediate and profound:

**Job Losses**: Hundreds of local residents lost stable employment. Many roles were specialized to institutional care, making reemployment difficult without retraining.

**Ripple Effects**: Local businesses—diners, shops, service providers—saw reduced foot traffic and revenue as hospital staff and visiting families disappeared.

**Housing and Infrastructure**: The sudden vacancy of such a massive campus created logistical and zoning challenges. Portions of the grounds were abandoned, while others required costly redevelopment.

**Identity Displacement**: For many families, Manteno wasn't just a job—it was a generational anchor. Its closure disrupted not only income but civic identity.

Lest we overlook this fact, Manteno Mental Health Center was a major employer within Kankakee County, and its closure represented a devastating blow to the regional workforce. While exact day-of-closure employment figures remain elusive—often buried in state archives or local newspaper accounts—it is documented that in 1983, Manteno housed 682 residents and employed 876 staff members. For decades, it stood as one of the largest single employers in the county, supporting hundreds—likely over a thousand—direct jobs at its operational peak.

These positions spanned a vast array of professions and skill levels:

**Medical and Clinical Staff**: Psychiatrists, psychologists, registered nurses (RNs), licensed practical nurses (LPNs), mental health technicians, social workers, occupational therapists, and physical therapists.

**Administrative and Professional Staff:** Managers, supervisors, clerical workers, human resources personnel, and financial administrators.

**Support Services**: Dietary staff (cooks, kitchen helpers), maintenance personnel (electricians, plumbers, HVAC technicians, groundskeepers), laundry workers, security guards, and transportation staff.

The sudden cessation of operations on December 31, 1985, meant the immediate termination of all these positions, throwing a significant portion of the local professional and working-class population into unemployment. For many, these were stable, well-paying state jobs with benefits—anchors of civic identity and economic security. Their loss was not just fiscal; it was ceremonial dislocation, a breach in the choreography of local life.

# ECONOMIC REALITIES

# AND RIPPLE EFFECTS OF THE CLOSURE

The economic shockwaves from the closure of Manteno Mental Health Center extended far beyond the immediate job losses, creating a cascade of destabilizing effects throughout Kankakee County and its surrounding communities.

**Massive Drain on Local Purchasing Power**: The cessation of salary and wage payments to hundreds of employees meant a sudden and severe outflow of spendable income. These were wages that had sustained local grocery stores, diners, gas stations, clothing shops, hardware stores, and service providers across Manteno, Kankakee, Bourbonnais, and Bradley. The loss of this consumer spending was not abstract—it was felt in empty booths, shuttered storefronts, and quiet registers.

**Negative Multiplier Effect**: Economists refer to the "multiplier effect," where each dollar earned is spent and re-spent within the local economy, generating additional activity. Manteno's closure inverted this principle. The initial job losses triggered reduced sales for local businesses, which in turn led to layoffs, reduced hours, and secondary job losses across the service and retail sectors. The economic choreography collapsed into silence.

**Erosion of the Local Tax Base**: Though state institutions like Manteno did not pay local property taxes, the loss of hundreds of employed residents indirectly impacted the tax base. Lower sales meant diminished sales tax revenues. Rising unemployment depressed property values, weakening school and municipal budgets. The fiscal rhythm faltered, and civic infrastructure absorbed the blow.

Manteno's closure was not just a bureaucratic decision—it was a ceremonial breach in the economic architecture of the region. The ledger didn't just lose numbers; it lost names, routines, and ensemble witness.

The closure of Manteno Mental Health Center triggered immediate strain on local social services. The sudden influx of hundreds of unemployed skilled and unskilled workers overwhelmed unemployment offices, food banks, and community assistance programs. Families accustomed to stable state incomes found themselves in need—stretching already limited resources thin. The safety net, designed for gradual hardship, was asked to absorb a mass dislocation.

Beyond the immediate crisis, Manteno's shutdown catalyzed a "brain drain" across Kankakee County. Highly specialized professionals—psychiatrists, psychologists, experienced nurses—faced limited opportunities for comparable employment within the region. Many were forced to relocate, taking with them not only their expertise but their civic presence, mentorship, and economic contribution. The community lost more than jobs—it lost institutional memory, ensemble wisdom, and the quiet choreography of care that had once anchored Manteno's corridors.

The rupture was not just fiscal—it was intellectual, emotional, and ceremonial. A keystone was removed, and the scaffolding of support trembled

The closure of Manteno Mental Health Center reverberated through the local housing market. The mass exodus of professionals seeking employment elsewhere—psychiatrists, nurses, administrators—combined with a broader economic downturn, led to a softening of demand for both rentals and home sales. Property values dipped, vacancies rose, and neighborhoods once sustained by institutional stability began to fray. The fiscal impact was measurable, but the emotional toll—felt in empty porches, quiet subdivisions, and "For Sale" signs that lingered—was harder to quantify.

More than an employer, Manteno was an anchor institution—a civic keystone woven into the fabric of Kankakee County for over five decades. It provided not only jobs, but identity, routine, and a steady pulse of economic and social engagement. Its absence left a void that was both economic and psychological. Residents lost not just income, but a sense of place. The rhythms of daily life—shift changes, cafeteria chatter, weekend visits—were disrupted. The closure was not merely administrative; it was a ceremonial severance from a shared narrative.

Manteno's silence became part of the landscape. And in that silence, the community was asked to reimagine itself without its keystone.

In essence, the closure of Manteno Mental Health Center was not merely the end of an institution—it was a profound economic catalyst that reshaped the contours of Kankakee County's economy. It underscored just how critical a single, large employer can be to the vitality and stability of a regional community. Quantifying its full financial impact would require careful historical economic analysis, but its significance as a job provider and economic engine cannot be overstated.

For long-serving employees, the closure presented a complex challenge. Many had accrued substantial tenure—decades of service, pension eligibility, and deep professional identity rooted in Manteno's corridors. In response, the State of Illinois offered redeployment opportunities within other state-run operations, including facilities under the Department of Mental Health and the Department of Corrections. Yet for many, relocation meant severance from community, disruption of family rhythms, and the loss of ensemble familiarity. The offer of continued employment, while technically sound, often failed to honor the ceremonial gravity of the breach.

Manteno's closure was not just a logistical pivot—it was a sovereign dislocation. And in its aftermath, the ledger of labor bore witness to more than numbers. It archived names, routines, and the quiet choreography of care that once sustained a county.

These placement options were primarily within existing state-run facilities that, while operational, were contending with persistent staffing shortages and high rates of employee turnover. Into this vacuum stepped former Manteno staff—individuals with deep institutional experience, procedural fluency, and ensemble wisdom. Their integration was not incidental; it was strategic. These facilities provided essential services to diverse and vulnerable populations, including individuals with physical disabilities, autism spectrum disorders, intellectual challenges, and co-occurring psychiatric diagnoses.

The redeployment of Manteno's workforce helped stabilize care environments that were stretched thin. Experienced nurses, aides, and therapists became anchors in systems struggling to maintain continuity. Their presence preserved not just quality of care, but the choreography of compassion—ritualizing routine, restoring dignity, and offering ensemble steadiness in facilities often marked by flux.

This was not merely workforce redistribution—it was mythic transference. Manteno's legacy did not vanish; it was refracted, carried forward in the hands and habits of those who had once walked its corridors.

This transition was far from seamless for the affected employees. A frequently encountered consequence of redeployment was the necessity of enduring significantly longer daily commutes. For many, the only viable alternative to these extended travels was the disruptive process of relocating their homes and families—uprooting children, severing community ties, and absorbing substantial financial strain. The burden was not just logistical; it was emotional, generational, and civic.

Beyond geography, employees faced the challenge of adapting to new work environments, unfamiliar organizational cultures, and distinct populations of individuals receiving services—including those with autism spectrum disorders, intellectual disabilities, and co-occurring psychiatric conditions. The adjustment demanded not only professional flexibility, but emotional endurance.

In situations where objective criteria for reassignment proved insufficient—particularly when tenure was equal or when informal networks threatened to skew opportunity—a unique and impartial system was implemented: a lottery. This mechanism, designed to ensure fairness and transparency, underscored the ceremonial gravity of the moment. Placement was no longer a matter of merit or preference—it was chance. And in that randomized choreography, Manteno's legacy was scattered across the state, refracted into new corridors, new routines, and new reckonings.

To maintain an unbiased selection process during Manteno's final phase, a unique and impartial system was implemented: the lottery. Individual slips of paper—each bearing an employee's name and pre-marked with either "yes" or "no" to ensure a predefined distribution of outcomes—were meticulously folded to conceal their contents. These slips were placed into a simple, unadorned straw bowl. One by one, employees drew their fate.

A "yes" designation meant the employee would either be redeployed to another role within the Manteno facility, if suitable positions remained, or continue in their current capacity until the institution's complete and final closure. These roles often involved wind-down operations, transitional care, or ceremonial duties tied to decommissioning.

The process was quiet, deliberate, and deeply symbolic. The straw bowl became a vessel of sovereign testimony. The folded slips, indistinguishable in form but decisive in consequence, ritualized the final choreography of Manteno's workforce. It was not just a drawing—it was a reckoning. And in that moment, each name became archive.

Conversely, a "no" designation signified a guaranteed offer of employment from the State of Illinois, facilitating a transition to an alternative position at a different state-operated facility or agency. This pathway typically included logistical support for relocation or reassignment, offering affected employees the opportunity to begin a new professional chapter outside of Manteno. For many, it ensured continuity of income and benefits—but at the cost of proximity, familiarity, and ensemble rhythm.

These reassigned roles spanned a range of institutions under the Department of Mental Health and the Department of Corrections, serving populations with diverse and complex needs. The transition was framed as smooth, but often felt abrupt. Employees were asked to carry their expertise into unfamiliar corridors, adapt to new organizational cultures, and reorient their care choreography to different institutional cadences.

The "no" slip did not mean dismissal—it meant dispersal. It was a sovereign dispatch, a ritualized redirection of Manteno's legacy into new geographies. And in that movement, the folded paper became archive, the straw bowl became compass, and each employee became a carrier of institutional memory.

I was one of many employees navigating a significant period of organizational restructuring within our department. When the results of the internal placement process were announced, my application for a preferred role was not approved—signaling a definitive "no" to my initial choice. That moment was more than professional disappointment; it was a ceremonial pivot.

In response, I was presented with three distinct alternative opportunities. Each demanded a considerable shift—not only in my professional focus, but in my daily logistics, my rhythm, and my sense of place. These options were not lateral. They were mythic recalibrations. They asked me to reimagine my role, my commute, and my choreography of care.

The process was framed as fair, but the emotional terrain was complex. Behind every "no" was a name, a routine, a hope. And behind every alternative was a reckoning—with geography, with identity, and with the quiet endurance required to begin again.

I was presented with three distinct alternatives—each a doorway, each a disruption.

The first was a position within the Department of Corrections, Juvenile Division, located in Aurora, Illinois. It would involve working directly with young people navigating the justice system—offering support, structure, and guidance in an environment shaped by accountability and reform.

The second was a management role at Howe Developmental Center in Tinley Park, an institution dedicated to individuals with developmental disabilities and intellectual challenges. This position would require overseeing operations and staff, ensuring high-quality care and programming in a setting defined by complexity and compassion.

The third was a role within a community-based psychiatric program in Chicago, focused on outpatient support for individuals with mental health needs. It promised less restriction, more autonomy, and a different cadence of care—one shaped by urban proximity and ensemble outreach.

Yet all three shared a common challenge: distance. Each required a daily commute exceeding an hour from my residence. The geography alone added weight to the decision—stretching time, reshaping routine, and demanding a recalibration of family rhythm and personal endurance.

These weren't just job offers. They were sovereign thresholds. Each asked me to reimagine my choreography of care, my proximity to home, and my place within a new institutional narrative. And in choosing, I wasn't just selecting a role—I was ritualizing a new chapter.

The finality arrived swiftly. Within a single year, the sprawling campus of Manteno Mental Health Center—once a vibrant, self-contained community dedicated to long-term psychiatric care—was officially closed. Its corridors, once echoing with the rhythms of institutional life, fell silent. But that silence did not linger. The industrious work of repurposing began almost immediately.

The vast complex, with its extensive grounds and numerous buildings, was meticulously transformed. Its new mission: to provide essential care, rehabilitation, and dignified housing for the brave men and women who had served our nation. On September 15, 1986, the doors officially opened to the Illinois Veterans' Rehabilitation Center at Manteno, breathing new life into structures that had once housed another vulnerable population.

The transition was not merely architectural—it was mythic. Manteno's legacy was reframed, its purpose re-choreographed. And in that reframing, the campus became a vessel of continuity, where care was not abandoned, but redirected. The walls remembered. The grounds bore witness. And the new mission honored both the past and the present in sovereign tandem.

This transition brought with it a stark numerical shift. In its final operational years leading up to the 1985 closure, Manteno Mental Health Center provided comprehensive, often long-term care for approximately 1,200 individuals experiencing severe mental health conditions. The facility employed a dedicated staff of around 700 professionals—psychiatric aides, nurses, therapists, medical personnel, administrative and support staff—all contributing to the intricate ecosystem of patient care and institutional management across its expansive campus.

In contrast, the newly established Illinois Veterans' Rehabilitation Center at Manteno, while offering invaluable services tailored to the unique needs of former service members, was designed to accommodate approximately 600 veterans, supported by a staff of roughly 450 individuals.

This represented a considerable reduction in both the number of persons served and the total employment opportunities within the Manteno campus. The shift was not just statistical—it was ceremonial. The rhythm of care was halved, the choreography of labor restructured, and the ensemble footprint compressed. Manteno's legacy was reframed, but its echo remained—carried in the corridors, remembered in the routines, and archived in the sovereign testimony of those who witnessed both eras.

Given the immense acreage of the campus—hundreds of acres that once offered space for therapeutic outdoor activities, vocational training, agricultural programs, and simply room to breathe and find solace—the question that continues to haunt many, myself included, is a profound and poignant one: Was it ever truly necessary to close Manteno Mental Health Center in its entirety?

Could a portion of its resources, its infrastructure, its staff expertise, and its unique therapeutic environment not have been preserved—perhaps even integrated with emerging models of community mental health care—rather than undergoing such a comprehensive dismantling?

The closure reflected a broader national trend toward deinstitutionalization, driven by evolving philosophies of care, increasing awareness of patient rights, and the promise of more localized, outpatient services. Yet for many who witnessed Manteno's operation firsthand, the closure felt like an irreversible loss—a forfeiture of a structured, large-scale environment that, despite its challenges and evolving practices, provided refuge and comprehensive support for a population often marginalized and underserved.

Manteno's grounds were not just acreage—they were choreography. They held the rhythms of long walks, vocational rituals, seasonal planting, and ensemble breath. And in their silence, we are left to wonder whether the promise of reform required the erasure of sanctuary.

But this narrative, at its heart, is not solely about my own career in mental health services, specifically within the hallowed—if sometimes challenging—halls of Manteno Mental Health Center. It is a profound and deeply personal testimony to the forgotten. To the distinct individuals whose lives intersected within those walls. To the complex and unique conditions they navigated with remarkable resilience.

Most importantly, it is a tribute to those extraordinary persons—both those receiving care and those providing it—who, through their vulnerability, their triumphs, and their profound human struggles, left an indelible mark on me and countless others who shared that time.

Many of those voices are now gone. Their stories fade with the passage of time. But their legacies endure—in the memories of those they touched, in the rhythms of care they helped choreograph, and in the sovereign testimony of those who still remember. Manteno was not just a facility. It was a constellation of lives. And this archive is for them.

# WORKING AT MANTENO

I arrived at Manteno Mental Health Center as a newly hired case worker—a role akin to what we'd now call a social worker, though the title barely captured the fluidity of the task. My duties were grounded in intake, assessment, "talk therapy," program planning, follow-up, and, if possible, discharge to another facility. But the real assignment was clear: I had been brought in to assist with the closure.

My job was to move people—human beings with histories, habits, and heartbreaks—into "less restrictive" environments. That phrase, so clean on paper, carried the weight of institutional unraveling. It meant evaluating whether someone who had lived within Manteno's rhythms for years could now be relocated to a group home, a community program, or a facility with fewer locks and more ambiguity.

On that first day, I walked the halls not as a visitor, but as a witness. The campus was vast, its architecture both imposing and tender. I met staff who had worked there for decades—nurses who knew every patient's nickname, aides who could read a mood from a shuffle, janitors who bore silent witness to every breach and breakthrough.

And I met patients—some lucid, some lost, all layered. Their stories weren't in the charts. They were in the routines, the gestures, the way they greeted me with suspicion or warmth. I was not there to fix them. I was there to move them. And that truth sat heavy.

The first intake I conducted was with a man named Leonard. He had been at Manteno for over twenty years. His diagnosis was. complex, but his handshake was firm He asked if I was "one of the closers." I said yes. He nodded, then said, "Then let's do it right."

That was my first day. Not a beginning, but a continuation. Not an assignment, but a reckoning. And from that moment on, every chart I opened felt like a ledger. Every discharge, a dispatch. Every silence, a sovereign testimony.

On my first day, before I'd even settled into the rhythm of intake forms or discharge planning, I was asked to supervise the cafeteria. The assignment was deceptively simple: ensure things moved in an orderly fashion from tray to table without violence or breach. It resembled a school lunchroom in structure, but not in psychology.

My added duty was to check the bathroom—specifically, to flush out the smokers. The door didn't open outward, but inward. I was told, without ceremony, that the safest procedure was to kick the door in before entering. Not for drama. For survival.

I did as instructed. The overcrowded bathroom erupted—smokers scurrying, cigarettes extinguished in haste, denials rehearsed mid-exhale. It was choreography born of routine breach.

Afterward, one gentleman approached me. He looked me over and asked, "Are you a rapist or a murderer?" I didn't know what to say.

You see, the psychology wasn't about credentials. It was about hierarchy of respect. Some patients respected violence. Some feared it. Some had learned to navigate institutions by decoding threat. It wasn't enough to say, "I'm neither." That answer lacked mythic weight.

In that moment, I understood: Manteno wasn't just a facility. It was a stage of sovereign roles, where every gesture was interpreted, every silence was read, and every new face had to earn its place in the ensemble.

I wasn't there to dominate. I was there to witness. And the cafeteria, on day one, became my first dispatch in the choreography of care

He hadn't seen me before. I was new. And in Manteno, newness was not neutral—it was a breach in the known choreography.

After the cafeteria cleared and the bathroom door settled back into its frame, he approached me. Calm. Direct. "Are you a rapist or a murderer?"

It wasn't a threat—it was a classification. A survival mechanism. A way to map the unfamiliar through a ledger of perceived danger.

I lied. I told him I was a murderer.

He smiled. "Welcome to Manteno," he said.

That was the ritual. That was the psychology. In a place where respect was often earned through mythic posture, where vulnerability could be dangerous and credentials irrelevant, I had entered the ensemble through narrative fit.

It wasn't about truth. It was about choreography. And in that moment, I understood: Manteno wasn't just a facility. It was a stage. And every role—staff, patient, witness—was cast through ritual, not résumé.

That afternoon marked a profound shift in me. I no longer saw "mental illness." I saw human beings.

These are the stories of some of these human beings with which I worked.

---

Later that afternoon, the sterile hum of the fluorescent lights in the unit seemed to amplify the silence. I found our lead psychologist, standing beside a gurney, its worn vinyl cushion waiting with a chilling patience. Beside him, a junior staff member, a man whose name I couldn't quite recall, stood ramrod straight, his expression unreadable. The air crackled with a peculiar tension, not hostile, but anticipatory, like the moment before a storm.

The psychologist turned to me, a glint in his eye that I couldn't decipher – wasn't quite amusement, wasn't quite malice, but something clinical and unnerving. "Ah, there you are," he said, his voice smooth, betraying none of the unit's underlying unease. "Perfect timing. We're ready to continue your training."

My gaze drifted to the gurney, then to the stack of thick leather straps neatly coiled on a nearby cart. My stomach tightened. Full leather restraints. I'd seen them in old documentaries, in sepia-toned photographs of institutions long since shuttered, but never in person. Certainly never at Manteno, not during my time.

"For today's exercise," he continued, gesturing towards the gurney with a sweep of his hand, "I want to place you in full leather restraints. It's an exercise in simulating the patient experience."

The words hung in the air, heavy and incongruous. Simulating the patient experience. My mind immediately flashed to the countless policy manuals, the endless training modules, the very ethos drilled into us from day one: Manteno prided itself on progressive, humane care. Restraints, especially full leather, were anathema to that philosophy. They were a relic.

"But," I began, the protest already forming on my tongue, "we don't use full leather restraints here. They've been explicitly phased out. They're considered..."

He held up a hand, cutting me off, his gaze unwavering. "Precisely. And for good reason. Full leather restraints were never used during my tenure at Manteno, nor yours. That practice, along with any form of such extreme physical limitation, had proven ineffective in managing behavior. It was an instrument to create compliance, yes, but more importantly, it was a tool to enforce an imbalance of power. A throwback, if you will, to the days when the hospital was severely understaffed, and compliance, not healing, was the primary goal."

His explanation, rather than assuaging my unease, deepened it. He was articulating the very arguments against the practice, yet proposing to enact it. The irony was a cold prickle on my skin. He was acknowledging the trauma, the ineffectiveness, the archaic nature of it all, only to then suggest I subject myself to it.

"Restraint, whether partial or full," he continued, as if reciting from a textbook, "has proven to be profoundly traumatic to the patient. It's not a 'learning' tool for them, but rather a source of fear, anger, and often re-traumatization. And as such, it is entirely ineffective in fostering any positive behavioral change or therapeutic alliance."

I swallowed hard, the contradiction a bitter taste in my mouth. If it was traumatic, ineffective, and not a learning tool for them, how could it be anything but traumatic and deeply contradictory as a "learning" tool for me? Was the lesson simply, "This is what it feels like to be powerless"? And if so, what kind of psychologist would deliberately inflict such a lesson, even in simulation?

The junior staff member stepped forward then, his face still carefully neutral, and picked up the first of the leather cuffs. The thick, oiled leather felt substantial, almost menacing. My heart hammered a warning against my ribs. To lie on that gurney, to expose myself to that manufactured vulnerability, under the guise of "training"... it felt less like education and more like an initiation into a darker, forgotten corner of institutional history.

The goal might have once been compliance, but in this moment, for me, it felt like an invitation to understand a kind of terror that Manteno had sworn it had left behind. The decision, though unspoken, was clear: participate, or fail to understand. And the thought of truly understanding, truly feeling that profound loss of control, was suddenly far more terrifying than I'd anticipated.

My agitation had been subtle, a quiet refusal to comply with the mandatory afternoon training. The psychologist, whose face was a roadmap of clinical indifference, had assessed my defiance as a prelude to escalation. His voice, measured and low, was the sound of a guillotine being sharpened.

"We need you to cooperate. We can do this the easy way, or we can deal with the consequences."

He didn't need to specify the consequences. They stood against the far wall, artifacts of institutional absolute power.

There was the gurney, the 'transport unit.' It was steel-framed, industrial grey, and utterly featureless save for the thick, black canvas straps coiled neatly beside its head. They were not just straps; they were harnesses designed to erase personhood, turning a man into a manageable object.

But, I wasn't agitated. Yes, I was. I was confused.

The psychologist did not acknowledge the distinction. He simply directed his gaze toward the gurney. "Let's get you settled now."

"No."

The word was quiet, definitive. It hung between us, heavier than the fluorescent light fixture humming above. I refused to lie on the gurney, to facilitate my own full restraint. The very act of climbing onto that cold metal slab felt like psychological suicide, a surrender not of force, but of essential self-respect.

He waited, his hands resting lightly on the padded counter, demonstrating an almost inhuman patience. He was expecting the resistance to break—either through exhaustion or through the sheer terror of what would happen if I forced his hand.

When I remained standing, merely tense but still contained, he adjusted his strategy.

"Then, perhaps a cooling-off period?" he suggested, his tone softening only marginally. "The timeout room is available. It will give you space to process this choice without further incident."

The timeout room. The 'Quiet Room,' as the brochures euphemistically called it. It was twenty feet down the corridor, behind a solid steel door with no handle on the inside. A soundproof box designed for sensory deprivation and absolute isolation.

I refused that too.

He sighed, the noise barely audible, the sound of a professional dealing with bureaucratic delays. He knew that forcing a full physical takedown in the main viewing corridor required paperwork and the involvement of two additional staff members. My refusal to cooperate had created an awkward stalemate. I was defiant, but not violent. I was resisting the procedure, not attacking the institution.

It was in that sustained, uncomfortable balance that the clarity struck me.

Just knowing those artifacts of institutionalization were present—the cold, ready gurney, the coiled restraints, the bolted, featureless door of the isolation room—was deterrent enough. It dictated every single micro-action I took.

When I spoke, I moderated my voice, keeping the pitch level. When I moved, I kept my hands visible and my movements slow, avoiding the sharp, sudden gestures that could be interpreted as a threat and trigger the institutional response protocol. My entire being was contained within the invisible boundary defined by the threat of those instruments. I was walking a tightrope stretched between my stubborn refusal and the immediate, crushing consequence of overstepping.

And then, it occurred to me that maybe that was the point.

The gurney was not primarily there for transport; it was a constant, stark reminder of the body's fragility and the ease with which it could be neutralized. The timeout room was not just for seclusion; it was the ultimate, concrete metaphor for being erased, defining the terror of non-existence within the system.

They didn't have to use the tools to control us. They just had to be visible.

The presence of the artifacts enforced compliance far more efficiently than their repeated deployment ever could. Every patient who had been here for more than a few days understood this unspoken contract. We weren't resisting the tools; we were resisting the path that led to the tools, maneuvering in the narrow, acceptable space granted to the "manageable" patient.

The psychologist didn't push me beyond the argument because he knew that as long as I could see the gurney and knew the seclusion room waited, I would temper my rebellion. I would provide him with the necessary minimum compliance required to avoid the final, dehumanizing step.

We were all dancers in a poorly lit room, carefully avoiding the tripwires.

I finally walked to the nearest chair and sat down slowly, deliberately. I had not surrendered, but I had submitted to the architecture of control.

The psychologist watched me, a flicker of professional satisfaction crossing his face. He didn't see my action as a calculated political move, only as the final capitulation of defiance.

He was wrong. It was the precise definition of the battleground.

I looked across the common room at a female patient, always quiet, always crocheting, her eyes wide and knowing. I saw the look of understanding in the dull gaze of young Michael, perpetually slumped on the couch. They were watching the interaction, gauging which lines could be safely crossed that day.

They knew. Every patient knew. The artifacts of institutionalization were not merely emergency mechanisms; they were monuments erected to silence, serving as the permanent, terrible boundary of our freedom. And their presence was the most powerful restraint of all.

---

The observation began the following day with a routine established by institutional mandate, evidenced by the formation of a queue. A line of patients waited, static and compliant. This daily ritual was the observable product of a token economy, a system implemented by the resident psychologist intended to structure positive and negative reinforcement for the population.

In this specific iteration of the economy, the "token" was not a symbolic currency or chip, but tangible funds. Patients stood in wait to receive their daily consequence, which manifested as either thirty-five cents ($.35) for documented "good" behavior or twenty-five cents ($.25) for documented "bad" behavior.

Crucially, the determination of behavior—good or bad—was based entirely on the presence or absence of a recorded incident report from the preceding twenty-four hours.

This structure immediately introduced a significant flaw in the mechanism of behavioral shaping. Because the consequence was delayed by a full day, it could not function as genuine immediate reinforcement. There was no connection between a patient's action in the moment and the subsequent reward or penalty. The only behavior actively shaped was the immediate one: standing in a long line to receive a delayed consequence tied to an outdated metric.

Furthermore, the scale of the differential made impact negligible. The entire spread between acceptable and unacceptable conduct was ten cents. That ten-cent difference was the established cost of a can of soda from the facility vending machine.

The outcome of the lengthy wait and the formalized system of delayed accountability was thus reduced to an administrative exercise. It was not consequence; it was an allocation of minimal funds based on documentation, perpetually divorced from the behavior it was purportedly designed to modify.

It was control, subtle and unquestioned and entirely meaningless – another artifact from the institutional days gone by.

The architecture of control was never just about objects. It was about the stories those objects silenced. Every patient who stood in that line, who moderated their gestures, who calculated the cost of a soda against the price of defiance—each carried a testimonial that the system could not quantify. The gurney, the timeout room, the ten-cent differential—they were not the story. They were the perimeter.

What follows are the voices that lived within that perimeter. Not case studies. Not diagnoses. But sovereign testimonials—fragments of ache, wit, and quiet rebellion. These are the patients I met. These are the stories Manteno tried to forget.

# MANTENO PATIENTS

# Kevin

The heavy door clanged shut, a sound that always felt final within those walls, sealing Kevin away from the world he'd just been torn from. The two officers, their faces unreadable, left without a backward glance, their boots echoing down the sterile hallway until silence reclaimed the space. "He's yours now," the officer's words hung in the air, a burden passed on, a responsibility cemented.

I looked at Kevin. Up close, the impression of a well-adjusted college student wavered, ever so slightly. His eyes, a startling clear blue, held a peculiar stillness. They didn't dart around the unfamiliar intake room, assessing, questioning, or betraying fear. Instead, they seemed to look through things, like a sheet of ice over deep, dark water. His posture was, indeed, impeccable, almost impossibly so, lending him a rigidity that felt less like confidence and more like a carefully constructed shell.

His composure was remarkable, almost unnerving. It wasn't the calm of someone who understood and accepted their situation, but the quietude of a lake before a storm, or perhaps, after one has already raged and passed, leaving only an eerie stillness in its wake. There was something in his very stillness that felt heavier, more potent, than any outward display of distress. It was the silence of a packed spring, ready to release its force. And I knew, with a certainty that settled deep in my stomach, that Kevin was going to be unlike any patient I had ever met before. The question wasn't what he had done, but what he would do, or perhaps, what he was truly thinking behind those impossibly clear blue eyes.

The days that followed folded into a quiet, unsettling routine of observation. Kevin remained a fixed point on the ward, a living statue amidst the ebb and flow of other patients – the anxious, the agitated, the melancholic. The Haldol, I knew, was a heavy-hitter, meant to break the catatonia, to unlock the rigid prison of his mind and body. Yet, for a long stretch, it seemed to have no discernible effect.

He would be gently guided to group therapy, his waxy arm lifted and placed, and he would stay, a silent, unmoving sentinel amongst the scattered chatter and occasional outbursts of others. He was there, yet profoundly absent. At meal times, a tray would be placed before him, and he would simply stare at it, his eyes tracking nothing, seeing nothing. Sometimes, a kind aide would spoon-feed him, and he would swallow, a purely physiological response, devoid of any apparent will or pleasure. It was like tending to a very complex, breathing doll.

My initial, dismissive thought of malingering had long since evaporated, replaced by a profound, unsettling awe. No one, not even the most skilled actor, could maintain such a state, such unyielding stillness, for so long without breaking. It was an exertion of will in reverse, a complete surrender to immobility. It was terrifying.

The stark facts of his file continued to haunt me in the quiet moments: the arson, the father's home, the impregnated girlfriend. Such brutal, human details, yet they felt so distant from the silent, inert man before me. Was this his way of coping? Of escaping an unbearable reality? Or was it simply the brain's ultimate short-circuit, a desperate attempt to shut down from an overwhelming onslaught? I had no answers, only questions that hung in the sterile air of the ward.

One afternoon, I sat charting nearby, feigning attention to my notes but covertly watching him. Kevin was standing by the window, as he often did, gazing out at the limited view of the hospital grounds. The sun cast a long shadow from his motionless form. A bird landed on the sill, chirped, and flew away. Kevin's gaze remained fixed. But then, something almost imperceptible happened. His eyelids, which had seemed glued open, fluttered. A micro-movement. A flicker of life in the unblinking stare.

I held my breath. Was it a side effect of the medication? A random twitch? Or... a nascent return?

Another week passed. The Haldol and Cogentin continued their work, a slow, chemical dance within his system. The doctor's notes spoke of "slow progress anticipated." But progress for Kevin was measured in millimeters, in the barest hints of agency. I found myself searching for these tiny signs, these fragments of the person locked within. It became a morbid game of 'Where's Waldo,' except Waldo was a flicker of life, a ghost in the machine.

The staff often talked about Kevin in hushed tones, marveling at his condition. Some found it creepy. Others, like me, found it profoundly sad. It was a stark reminder of how fragile the human mind could be, how easily it could break and retreat into an impenetrable fortress. The medication was working, albeit agonizingly slowly. The charts now indicated a slight decrease in muscle rigidity, a fractional improvement in eye following. But to the untrained eye, Kevin was still Kevin – the statue.

Then, one evening, as the ward was quieting down, I witnessed something truly new. Kevin was standing by his bed, arms still at his side, his posture familiar. But his head, which had been perfectly level for weeks, tilted. Just a fraction of an inch, to the left. He held it there for a moment, the movement slow, deliberate, almost painful to watch. Then, just as slowly, he straightened it again. It was not a reflex. It was not a side effect. It was an action.

It was the first time I had witnessed him initiate a movement that wasn't a biological imperative like swallowing. It was a spark. A tiny, fragile spark in the vast, dark chamber of his catatonia.

I felt a surge of something – not hope, exactly, but a deep, quiet recognition. The man was still in there. He was still fighting, or perhaps, simply, returning. And I was there to witness it, a silent observer to a silent battle. The conversation was still absent, but the story, I realized, was just beginning to unfold.

The fluorescent hum of the psychiatric ward was the soundtrack to my days. I was his case worker. My presence was part of the intricate, often silent, rhythm of the place. There was no conversation, no expectation of it, especially not with Kevin. When I first saw him, he was a statue. Catatonic. Eyes open, unseeing, fixed on some unbreachable point in a world only he inhabited. He was there, breathing, a body occupying space, but the person held within was utterly absent.

The shift, when it came, was a slow, gradual unfolding, then an astonishing acceleration. Within two weeks, the stillness began to crack. Kevin was actively moving around, his long limbs no longer frozen in place. He started to speak, his voice scratchy from disuse, but willing to engage. He'd talk to me, answer my quiet questions, but his face... his face was a constant glare. A fierce, unwavering intensity that seemed to bore into the very air around him, a silent, internal scream made visible.

It took time, and the subtle cues of his increasing, if still guarded, trust, to understand that this glare wasn't directed at me, or at the sterile walls, or even at the distant, muted world beyond the hospital window. It was fixed on the voices in his head.

Those voices were, as he eventually confided in hushed, fragmented sentences, "extremely aggressive and negative." He'd grip the arms of his chair, knuckles white, his eyes darting as if trying to pinpoint the invisible speakers. "They tell me I'm a bad person," he whispered, his voice cracking with the effort. "The worst. They say I should die. They want me to die." The voices were relentless, a ceaseless cacophony of condemnation, dissecting his past actions, chastising him for every perceived failing, every misstep. They were the ultimate prosecutors, the final, unforgiving judges.

And in their relentless, internal judgment, I heard an echo. A chilling, painful resonance of the world outside. Kevin, I eventually learned, carried the legal status of NGRI – Not Guilty by Reason of Insanity. The voices in his head, these cruel, unwavering tormentors, articulated precisely the societal judgment that often clung to such a verdict.

They told him he was guilty, that he had committed unforgivable acts, and that while he might have "skirted accountability" in the legal sense because of his mental illness, he was still fundamentally, irredeemably flawed. The voices were a psychic manifestation of that lingering accusation, that deep-seated belief that mental illness was merely an excuse, not a devastating truth. They were the world's harsh verdict, amplified a thousandfold; an eternal, inescapable echo within his own mind. And I, but simply a witness, could only listen, and silently bear the weight of his profound, internal agony.

The sterile hum of the fluorescent lights in the ward always seemed to follow me, a constant, low-level thrum against the backdrop of whispers and distant shouts. As a caseworker in this psychiatric hospital, I navigated a world where reality bent and fractured, where hope was as fragile as a thin pane of glass. Kevin was one of those windows, and his story was one I carried close.

I'd been his caseworker since his admission, a quiet young man haunted by the shadow of an arson he'd committed. For weeks, he'd mostly kept to himself, a silent, watchful presence. But gradually, a month or so into his stay, cracks of light began to appear. He started to nod when addressed, then offered brief, polite answers. Eventually, I even saw him smile – a fleeting, almost shy curve of lips that hinted at a softer person beneath the layers of his illness.

Noting this progress, I called him to my office, the small space smelling faintly of old coffee and institutional cleaner. He sat across from me, hands clasped on his knees, an openness in his posture I hadn't seen before.

"Kevin," I began, "how would you feel about earning some money while you're here?"

His eyes, usually downcast, flickered up, a spark of curiosity in their depths. He agreed, a soft 'yes' barely audible. I also broached the idea of GED courses, something we offered to help patients prepare for life outside. He seemed interested initially, but that ambition quickly faded. It became clear, after a few sessions, that Kevin was functionally illiterate. The GED was a mountain he couldn't yet fathom. A job, tangible and immediate, meant far more to him.

I referred him to the hospital workshop, a place that provided supervised employment to patients. His task: sorting silverware for the cafeteria. It was repetitive, simple work, but it was work. Each day he returned from the workshop, I'd ask him how it went. And each day, he'd offer that small, emerging smile.

"I'm the fastest worker there," he'd tell me, a quiet pride in his voice. "Looking forward to my first check."

His demeanor softened noticeably. He never denied the arson when it came up in therapy, a somber memory he carried, but now he seemed on the verge of hopefulness. He had a job. More importantly, the tormenting voices that had plagued him for so long had shifted. They were still present, a constant companion in his mind, but they now told him different things. "Good things," he'd say. "They tell me I'm a handsome young man. That I look good. That I'm working." The voices, once insidious and destructive, had mirrored his external success, offering affirmations instead of condemnations. It was a fragile peace, but it was peace.

Then came payday.

Kevin approached my office, not with the usual hopeful glint, but with a stiff, almost rigid posture. He pushed open the door and stood before my desk, the small envelope clutched in his hand.

"I quit," he said, the words flat.

I stared at him, bewildered. "Quit? Kevin, why? You were doing so well. You said you were the fastest worker."

He didn't answer immediately. Instead, he slowly, deliberately, pulled the piece of paper from the envelope and laid it on my desk. It was his paycheck. Two weeks of work, sorting countless forks, spoons, and knives. Two weeks of waking up with purpose, finding pride in effort, hearing kinder voices.

The total printed on the slip: $16.

Sixteen dollars. For two weeks of his time, his effort, his burgeoning hope.

Some might argue that $16 was better than nothing. I suppose a penny is better than nothing too. But to Kevin, it wasn't about the absolute value. It was an insult. He hadn't expected to get rich working in the hospital workshop; he understood the constraints. But two weeks of consistent, dedicated labor, only to be handed such a paltry sum, utterly deflated him. It stripped away the nascent pride he'd cultivated. It diminished his effort.

I looked at the check, then back at Kevin's face, now devoid of that shy smile. There was no anger, just a deep, quiet disappointment. I didn't try to talk him out of it. I'd learned over the years that this wasn't an isolated incident. Many patients were insulted by the low pay, a system that sometimes inadvertently devalued their attempts at self-worth and independence. For Kevin, $16 wasn't a reward; it was a stark reminder of how little his efforts were deemed worth. And in a mind already wrestling with its own fragmented reality, that message could be devastating.

The day of discharge arrived with little fanfare, as most things did on the ward. Kevin woke, dressed meticulously in an outfit he'd carefully pressed himself – a crisp blue shirt, neatly creased trousers. He ate breakfast, exchanged pleasantries with the nursing staff, and packed the few belongings he had: his hospital-issued toiletries, a worn paperback, the pamphlets I'd given him neatly folded in a plastic bag. There was no family waiting, no enthusiastic farewell committee. Just a quiet handover of paperwork, a final signature, and the opening of a heavy door.

I stood by the nurses' station, watching him go. He walked with a confident gait, head held high, looking every inch the capable, put-together man the psychiatrist had signed off on. He turned at the end of the hallway, offered a small, almost imperceptible nod in my direction, and disappeared around the corner. The silence he left behind felt heavier than any noise. It was the sound of an absence. A successful discharge, by all medical standards. And yet, a hollow victory.

I called the number Kevin had given me for his friend, a habit born of years of experience and countless empty promises. It rang three times before an answering machine kicked in – a generic male voice, no name. I left a brief message, identifying myself and asking if I could confirm Kevin's arrival. No call back. I tried again the next day. Still nothing. A knot tightened in my stomach. Hope, even a fragile one, was a dangerous thing in this line of work.

A week later, Kevin called me. His voice was calm, almost devoid of emotion, a stark contrast to the bright, agreeable patient who'd left the ward. "It didn't work out with my friend," he said, the words carefully chosen, without inflection. "He... had other plans." No anger, no despair. Just a simple statement of fact, as if describing the weather. He was calling from a public phone, he explained. He didn't have a phone himself. He was staying in a shelter – one of the referrals I'd given him, a small mercy. He'd followed through on that at least. He sounded tired. Not clinically depressed, not agitated, but simply tired. The kind of exhaustion that comes from navigating a world not built for you, even when you're functionally 'better.'

I arranged for an emergency follow-up appointment, my heart sinking with each word. Kevin was still taking his medication, still well-groomed, still polite. He described his days: applying for minimum wage jobs, walking miles between interviews and the shelter, eating pre-made meals. He was doing everything 'right' according to the pamphlets, the therapy, the societal expectations. But the spark, the anomalous composure that had charmed the ward, seemed to have dimmed. It wasn't a relapse into psychosis, but a quiet, creeping disillusionment. The outside world, for Kevin, was just a larger, more complex institution, where the rules were unwritten and the support structures invisible. And I, his case worker, was still navigating the labyrinth with him, one phone call, one referral, one quiet observation at a time.

The administrator pursed his lips. "An alibi, you say? And you believe him, Brian?" His tone was less accusatory of me, and more a weary skepticism born of years in the system. "The police will want to speak to this friend. And to Kevin, of course."

And then he sat back in his chair and stated, "Welcome to mental health."

I felt a familiar knot tighten in my stomach. This wasn't merely about Kevin; it was about the hospital's reputation, my professional judgment, and, most importantly, Kevin's fragile grasp on the outside world. An accusation like this, even unfounded, could send him spiraling.

"I have no reason not to believe him," I said, trying to keep my voice steady. "He sounded genuine, and he offered the information freely. I'll follow up with him immediately. I can also try to reach the friend, if you'd like me to relay their contact information to the police."

The administrator nodded, already moving on to other pressing matters. "Just make sure we're cooperating fully, and that we have all our ducks in a row. These situations can get messy."

Messy. That was an understatement.

I hung up, the phone feeling heavy in my hand. My mind raced. Kevin had sounded calm when he called, almost detached as he relayed the rumors, but that was often his way of coping with stress. Below the surface, I knew he'd be churning. The accusation alone would be a massive trigger for his paranoia, which we had worked so hard to manage during his stay.

My first call was to Kevin. He answered on the second ring, his voice still flat. "It's me, Brian," I said. "I just spoke with the hospital administrator. He's aware of the arson accusation. Have the police contacted you yet?"

"No," he said. "Not directly. Just... people are talking. Whispering. My landlord looked at me funny this morning."

"Right. Look, about your friend. Can you give me his name and number? It would be helpful if I could speak to him, or at least pass his information on to the police so they can confirm your alibi."

There was a pause. A long, uncomfortable pause. "Kevin?" I prompted, a chill snaking down my spine. "He's... his name is Mark," Kevin finally said, his voice softer, slightly hesitant. "He... he works nights. He was home. We were playing video games."

"And he's willing to confirm that?"

"He said he would," Kevin replied, but the conviction in his voice seemed to have wavered. "He's... a good friend."

The pause, the slight hesitation, the change in tone – it was subtle, but I knew Kevin well enough to pick up on it. It wasn't the confident 'yes' he'd given me yesterday. It was laced with a fragile hope, perhaps even a plea.

I thanked him and told him I'd be in touch. My gut instinct was screaming at me. A perfectly solid alibi doesn't come with that kind of emotional whitespace. I found myself doubting, just a little, for the first time since this whole thing began. What if there was more to it? What if "Mark" wasn't as willing to corroborate as Kevin believed, or as he wanted me to believe?

I spent the next hour trying to track down Mark. Kevin hadn't given me a number, just a general 'friend in the building' description. It was clear Kevin didn't want me digging too deep, or perhaps he didn't have the contact information readily available himself. This lack of concrete detail only amplified my unease.

Later that afternoon, two officers from the local precinct arrived at the hospital. They were polite but firm. They wanted to know everything about Kevin's discharge, his history, any recent triggers, any tendencies.

"He has no history of violence or arson," I stated emphatically, pulling up his file. "His primary diagnosis is schizophrenia, managed well with medication. We've focused on social integration, coping mechanisms for paranoia, and establishing a support network. There's nothing in his record to suggest he's capable of this."

One officer held up a hand. "We understand that. But a fire was set at the old, abandoned textile mill last night, just a few blocks from where Kevin was discharged. There are witnesses who saw someone fitting his general description in the vicinity. And we've learned he has a history of fascination with fire, specifically controlled fires, from an incident years ago that didn't lead to charges, but raised flags during an earlier psychiatric evaluation."

My blood ran cold. Fascination with fire? Why wasn't that prominently flagged in his current file? Had it been a minor note in an old report, overlooked during intake? I felt a wave of professional inadequacy, quickly followed by a fierce determination to protect Kevin.

"That 'fascination' was years ago, when he was much younger and experiencing a severe un-medicated episode," I countered, though internally I was scrambling. "He's stable now. He's not that person anymore."

"He told you he has an alibi?" the officer asked, leaning forward. "With a friend named Mark?"

"Yes," I confirmed, "he said he was at his friend's apartment. He said Mark would corroborate."

"We'll be speaking to Kevin and his friend directly," the officer concluded, standing up. "We just wanted to get your initial assessment and understand the context of his recent discharge. We appreciate your cooperation."

As they left, a sense of dread washed over me. The old textile mill. The "general description." The forgotten detail about fire. And Kevin's hesitant alibi. All the pieces were fitting together in a way that terrified me, not just for Kevin, but for the fundamental trust I had placed in his recovery, and in my own ability to guide him. The line between reality and his internal struggles suddenly felt dangerously thin, and I was on the precipice, bracing for the fall.

Turns out Kevin was telling the truth. No charges filed. It was someone else. And that's what mattered in that moment. Someone else.

I sat with the file open, the administrator's voice still echoing, the officers' questions still lingering. But Kevin's voice—flat, hesitant, honest—was the one I carried. He hadn't spiraled. He hadn't lied. He had endured. And in this line of work, that was everything.

# Garnett

"I have five billion brothers, Brian."

Garnett was the most joyful and most delusional man in the hospital. He had lived there more than twenty years. With a build and walk similar to Red Foxx, Garnett was more than happy. He was joyful. Everyday. Within these walls he lived in comfort, filled with laughter though he never cracked a joke. No. He just laughed at other people's jokes. And sometimes, nothing at all.

He had no known family or friends. He was alone in every sense of the word. But he declared he had five billion brothers. He not only declared it, but it was also a constant in his rhythmic joy. Pressed for specifics, he would tell you that among his five billion brothers were Walter Payton, the entire Bears football team, Mike Ditka, Gayle Sayers, Martin Luther King, Jr. and anyone else's name one might throw into the conversation. "Yep. Yep. I know them all. They're my brothers."

No sisters? "Naw."

He watched baseball games on television. Usually, the Chicago Cubs when WGN was a mainstay on television. They, too, were his brothers. And the fans in the park. When the camera panned over the crowd, and the crowd waved at the camera, Garnett waved at the crowd.

He waved with a sincerity that knew no bounds, a genuine connection forged in the ether of his own vibrant reality. To Garnett, those roaring stadium crowds weren't anonymous faces; they were kin, flesh and blood in spirit, cheering alongside their shared brothers on the field. The announcers, the umpires, the occasional politician glimpsed on the news – all fell under the vast umbrella of his fraternal network.

His laughter, a deep, resonant rumble, was a permanent fixture in the common room. It wasn't a boisterous, attention-grabbing laugh, but an ever-present hum of contentment that would erupt fully when someone else made a comment, or sometimes, when he simply caught sight of an image on the television screen that only he fully understood. A commercial for a car, a weather report, even the static between channels could elicit a chuckle, as if the universe itself were sharing a private joke with him.

Staff and patients alike became accustomed to Garnett's unwavering good spirits. He never asked for anything, never complained, never seemed to experience a moment of sadness or anger. His needs were simple, and his joy was absolute. When a new person joined the ward, they might initially find his persistent cheer unsettling or even unnerving. But soon enough, Garnett's presence became like the hospital's clock, a reliable, constant tick of pure, unadulterated happiness. He was a man suspended in a singular, perfect moment, eternally surrounded by billions of brothers and an unending stream of shared laughter, all within the quiet, contained world of the hospital walls.

The ward had a hum to it, a low, constant thrum of fluorescent lights, hushed footsteps, and the distant clink of medication trolleys. Identities often felt like they blurred in there, stripped down to diagnoses, routines, and the shared, unspoken anxiety that permeated the air. We were patients, and sometimes, it felt like that label overshadowed everything else we were or had been.

Then there was him.

He even looked the part, though what "the part" was, I couldn't quite say – perhaps the part of simple, unburdened joy. Smiling, bright-eyed, he'd move through the common room, or past us in the corridor, and without fail, he would greet us. Not with a generic "hello," or a nod, but by name.

"Brian," he'd say, his voice clear and genuinely cheerful. And that was all.

And that was his superpower.

It sounds small, almost trivial, but in that sterile, often depersonalizing environment, it was monumental. Many of us struggled to string together coherent thoughts, let alone connect with others. Days could merge into one another, marked only by meal times and therapy sessions. To be individually singled out, to have your name – your fundamental identifier – remembered and spoken with warmth, was a jolt of pure humanity.

I watched others react. The withdrawn woman who rarely made eye contact would sometimes offer a fleeting, almost imperceptible smile in return. The man who often stared blankly at the wall would turn his head, a flicker of recognition in his eyes. For a moment, we weren't just patients in a hospital gown. We were a person, distinct and acknowledged.

He didn't ask probing questions, didn't offer advice. He simply saw us. He didn't seem to notice the tremors in one person's hands, or the distant stare in another's eyes. He only saw the person behind it, and he honored that person by speaking their name.

His memory was flawless. He knew every single person on the ward, staff and patients alike, and he knew them by name. It wasn't a performance; it was just how he was. He moved through his own struggles, whatever they might have been, with this extraordinary capacity for simple, direct connection.

For me, hearing my name from him was like a small anchoring line thrown into turbulent waters. It reminded me I was still me, despite the fog and the fear. It was a brief, powerful affirmation that I hadn't been entirely subsumed by illness or environment. He didn't try to fix us, didn't try to understand our complex histories. He just remembered our names, and in doing so, he reminded us of our own. That simple act, in that place, was a profound and enduring gift.

The fluorescent hum of the ward was a constant companion, a low-frequency drone that became part of the background noise of my days. As a caseworker in a psychiatric hospital, my hours were a tapestry woven with assessments, group sessions, medication rounds, and the sometimes heartbreaking, sometimes baffling stories of the people entrusted to our care. It was a demanding landscape, and every small win, every flicker of connection, felt like a vital breath of fresh air.

Garnett was one of those breaths, though his approach was always the same, delivered with a polite, almost formal tilt of his head. "Brian," he'd begin, his voice a gravelly murmur, "I need to talk to you in your office?"

This routine played out at least four times a week. Initially, in my greener days, I'd brace myself. I'd think, This is it. A breakthrough. A revelation about his history, perhaps a flicker of lucidity that will illuminate a path forward. I'd mentally review his file, preparing for a deep dive into the labyrinth of his mind, hoping to unearth a piece of the puzzle that was Garnett.

But it was never that.

"No," was the simple reality of it. Asking to speak to me in my office was code. Code for a brief, sacred ritual that had nothing to do with therapy or breakthroughs, and everything to do with humanity. It was code for three cigarettes.

We'd walk down the corridor, past the nurses' station, past the day room where the television droned, and into the small, utilitarian space I called my office. The door would click shut, not locked, but firm enough to create a bubble of quiet distinct from the ward. Garnett would settle into the worn armchair opposite my desk, a sigh of contentment escaping him as he sank into its relative comfort.

I'd offer him the pack, and he'd carefully extract three, placing them on the desk like precious gems. I'd light the first for him, the small flame momentarily illuminating the deep lines etched around his eyes. He'd inhale, a long, slow draw, and then exhale a plume of smoke that, for a few blissful seconds, obscured the sterile white walls.

We rarely spoke of his diagnosis, or his treatment plan, or even the incidents that had brought him to us. Instead, we talked – or rather, he talked, and I listened, sometimes offering a prompt or a shared chuckle – about everything and nothing. He'd comment on the quality of the hospital coffee, compare it unfavorably to a brew he remembered from "the outside," or speculate on the true meaning of the hospital's bland, rotating menu. He'd tell me about a strange dream he'd had, or a particularly amusing bird he'd seen outside the window. Sometimes, the "nonsense" was simply a series of non-sequiturs, weaving from the weather to a snippet of a song he'd heard, to a memory of a distant relative he barely knew.

And we would laugh. It wasn't always uproarious, side-splitting laughter, but often a quiet, shared amusement. A gentle meeting of two minds over the absurdity of a situation, the simple pleasure of a cigarette, or the sheer, unbridled silliness of a thought. It was laughter that cut through the clinical veneer, that momentarily erased the roles of patient and caseworker, leaving only two people sharing a moment of respite.

In those brief, smoky interludes, away from the watchful eyes of the ward, away from the constant demands and often profound sadness, Garnett wasn't just a patient on a chart. He was a man with a wry sense of humor, a peculiar observational style, and an undeniable need for a small, consistent slice of normalcy.

It was nonsense, yes. It wasn't therapy in any traditional sense. But it was human connection, pure and unadulterated. And in the sometimes-overwhelming reality of my work, that nonsense, those three cigarettes, and those shared laughs were more than just welcome; they were essential. They were the small, resonant reminders that behind every diagnosis, there was always, always, a person yearning to simply be seen, and heard, and understood, even if just for a few fleeting minutes over a shared puff of smoke.

Then, one day, a nurse called me. She told me Garnett had punched one of the other nurses. I was shocked. Garnett had never demonstrated violence or anger. Oh, sometimes he grumbled, but it passed.

I walked to the nurse's station, nodded to Garnett. The nurse stated, "This man tells us every day he has five billion brothers. We can't reinforce these delusions."

Garnett slinked off to sit on the sofa. I looked at the nurse and leaned in quietly. She continued, "So, I told him he doesn't have five billion brothers. He has no family that we know of. And then he hit me." She pointed to her bleeding nose for emphasis.

I entered the nurse's station – a sacred place where the nurses dispensed medication and demands no patient could meet. I said, simply, "If Garnett says he has five billion brothers, he has five billion brothers."

The nurse stared at me, her hand still hovering over her bloody nose, mouth agape. "Brian, are you hearing yourself? We're here to treat delusions, not encourage them! He just assaulted me because of this nonsense!"

"He assaulted you, yes," I conceded, my voice still low, "but not because of nonsense. He assaulted you because you told him his family didn't exist. Imagine someone telling you your entire family was a lie, a figment of your imagination. How would you react?"

Her anger flared, eclipsing the shock. "We are professionals here! We can't just let patients live in fantasy land!"

"We're here to provide care," I countered, looking past her, out at Garnett who sat on the sofa, hunched, a small, defeated figure. "And sometimes, care means understanding that a person's reality, however different from ours, is still their reality. It's the framework they live in. When you dismantle that, you dismantle them."

I walked out of the station, leaving the nurse fuming. I approached Garnett slowly, giving him space. He didn't look up, just kept staring at his hands. I sat a little distance from him on the sofa, not too close, not too far.

"Garnett," I said, my voice soft, almost a whisper.

He flinched, then slowly, hesitantly, met my gaze. His eyes, usually clouded with an inner distance, held a raw, exposed vulnerability.

"Your brothers," I continued, "are they around today?"

A flicker of something—relief, perhaps, or a fragile spark of hope—crossed his face. He nodded, almost imperceptibly. "They're... they're always around, Brian." His voice was barely audible, raspy from disuse and recent distress. "Always."

"That's good," I said, simply. "Family is important, Garnett."

He finally looked at me fully, a faint, almost imperceptible easing of the tension in his shoulders. He didn't say anything more about his brothers, or the nurse, or the punch. But for a moment, in that shared, silent understanding, I felt a connection, a small repair in the fragile fabric of his world. It wasn't about five billion, or one, or none. It was about respect for the world he inhabited, and the pain of having it denied. And sometimes, in a place like this, that was the only medicine that truly mattered.

Garnett never asked us to believe. He asked us to listen. To wave back. To remember his name. And when the ward forgot, when the archive denied his brothers, he flinched. But when I asked, softly, if they were still around, he said yes. Always. And I believed him.

# Louie

Every morning, the hospital hummed to a peculiar, yet comforting, rhythm. The fluorescent lights flickered to life, the smell of institutional coffee mingled with disinfectant, and the soft clatter of breakfast trays began. And every morning, without fail, my day truly started when I walked into the dining hall.

Louie was always there, already seated at his usual spot by the window, a cup of lukewarm tea before him and a half-eaten muffin on his plate. He was an elderly gentleman, his face a roadmap of wrinkles, his hands gnarled but still capable of a firm grip. He claimed he once played minor league baseball for the Chicago Cubs. At least, that was his story. Who was I to deny him that reality? Maybe he did. Maybe he didn't. If Louie said so, he did. It was a truth he carried with him, a worn but cherished photograph in his mind.

And so it was that every morning when I arrived at work, Louie would look up, his eyes, though a little faded, still holding a spark. He'd declare, with the unwavering conviction of an umpire calling a home run, "The Cubs won the World Series!" That was all. A simple declaration of truth that Louie brought forth every single day, regardless of the season, the weather, or the actual standing of the Chicago Cubs. It was his anchor, a buoy bobbing in the tumultuous sea of his memory, tethering him to a glorious, if perhaps imagined, past.

Next to him sat Mary, another elderly patient. Her hair, once a vibrant silver, was now a wispy cloud around her head, and her gaze often drifted to some unseen horizon. She was part of Louie's ensemble, an unwitting, yet essential, participant in his daily ritual. For when Louie declared victory, Mary would invariably smile, a soft, almost ethereal expression, and murmur, "Such a pretty bird at the window."

Louie would look at Mary then, a flicker of irritation, or perhaps just habit, crossing his face. "Shut up," he'd grumble, not unkindly, but with the weary resignation of a man who'd heard the same interjection a thousand times.

Mary, unfazed, would counter, her voice as light as a feather, "Such a pretty bird."

Every day. Like clockwork. This was the rhythm that began my workday at the hospital. I'd nod to Louie, offer Mary a quiet "Good morning," and then continue my rounds, carrying the echo of their voices with me. The Cubs had won, and a pretty bird was at the window. And in that small, certain truth, there was a kind of peace.

So it was that year I had worked both Christmas Eve and Christmas Day, trying to fill in some family time. The next day, I was exhausted. And then I heard Louie. "The Cubs won the World Series today."

Exhaustion can make a person say and do almost anything. Certainly, it's not an ally. I said, "Louie, it's the day after Christmas. No one plays baseball in the winter."

Then, I caught myself and braced myself behind a thin partition.

The pool balls thudded against the thin partition, chipped paint spraying from the particle board. I pressed myself against it, heart thumping, the exhaustion suddenly burned away by a jolt of pure adrenaline. Louie was a big man, and when he went, he went. His shouts were a guttural, raw sound, peppered with more obscenities about baseball and my parentage. This wasn't a playful tantrum; this was a full-blown psychotic break, triggered by... what? The Christmas cheer? The lack of baseball?

Through the din, Mary's voice, light and almost melodic, cut through the aggression. "Such a pretty bird," she repeated, closer now. I risked a peek around the edge of the partition. Louie was still by the pool table, arms windmilling as he roared at a phantom umpire, but Mary was standing a few feet from him, looking intently at the blank wall beside the dartboard, a faint smile playing on her lips. She seemed utterly oblivious to the projectiles or the rage.

My first priority was safety. Mine, Louie's, and anyone else in the dayroom. I scanned the room quickly. Fortunately, it was early, and most of the other patients were still in their rooms or the dining hall. Just one other patient, old Mr. Henderson, was in a corner chair, head bowed, seemingly lost in his own world, or perhaps just wisely ignoring the chaos. No immediate targets for Louie other than myself and the rapidly disappearing pool balls.

I needed to get help. I took a deep breath, trying to project a calm I didn't feel. "Louie," I called out, my voice as steady as I could make it, "Let's take a break, okay? The Cubs will play again next season." Wrong move. He roared, picked up another ball, and hurled it with surprising force. It missed me by a foot, shattering against the glass of a picture frame on the far wall. The sound was sharp, final.

I didn't try talking again. I knew the drill. De-escalation wasn't an option when he was this far gone. I edged my way towards the emergency call button by the nurses' station, keeping the office partition between me and Louie's line of fire. My fingers fumbled slightly as I pressed it, the familiar shrill beep echoing through the halls, a summons for help, a signal that peace had indeed shattered.

Mary, meanwhile, continued her surreal monologue. "Yes, a lovely blue. And the song... so sweet." She seemed to be having a perfectly pleasant, if entirely private, conversation with an invisible companion, a serene counterpoint to Louie's violent crescendo. It was a typical morning in the unit, just with a little more shattered glass than usual, and a lot more tired Brian.

That morning, the usual quiet before the full rush of the day was punctuated by the sound of office doors opening and closing quickly – my colleagues starting their rounds, their voices hushed but busy. Then, Ed, my supervisor, emerged from his office, his gait deliberate as he approached the common area.

"Louie," Ed began, his voice clear, "The Cubs won the World Series."

Louie, a man of quiet habits and a contemplative gaze, paused mid-bite from his breakfast. He looked up, his eyes searching Ed's face, trying to ascertain if this improbable news was serious. Ed, sensing his doubt, elaborated with a slight, almost imperceptible nod. "The Cubs won. They swept... the Cardinals."

That was enough for Louie. The impossible had been made real, at least for this morning. He nodded slowly, a small, private victory registered in his expression, and then calmly resumed eating his breakfast. The world, in that moment, had aligned for Louie.

I was across the room, gathering pool balls, placing them back into the rack, preparing for the day's activities. I heard Ed's voice again, this time directed at me. "Brian, come see me in my office." I slowed my movements, stacking the colored spheres with more care than necessary. Mary, another patient, sat by the window, entirely absorbed in her own world. "Such a pretty bird," she murmured, pointing vaguely at the empty sill outside, her voice soft and entirely unconcerned with the baseball triumph or my supervisor's summons. She often found beauty where others saw none.

I eventually finished gathering the balls and walked towards Ed's office, feeling the familiar weight of exhaustion that often settled on me even before the day had truly begun. I pushed open his door, stepped inside, and sat down in the visitor's chair. My shoulders sagged a little.

Ed leaned back in his own chair, a bemused smile playing on his lips, a look I knew well. "What did you learn today, Brian?" he asked, his tone gentle, probing.

I looked at him, the irony of the question not lost on me, nor on him. I understood what he was asking, the deeper layer of observation he expected. But today, my answer was simple, direct, and laden with the truth of the daily cycles we witnessed. "The Cubs won the World Series," I stated, my voice flat. Then, unable to resist the edge of weariness and the strange, repetitive nature of our reality, I added, "They always win the World Series. Every damn day the Cubs win the World Series, Ed."

Ed chuckled, a quiet, understanding sound. He didn't need to say anything more. He just nodded, a slight inclination of his head, and then dismissed me. I knew he understood.

The next morning, I came to work, pushing through the doors into the perpetual hum of the hospital. I saw Louie in his usual spot, eating breakfast. I saw Mary at the window, her gaze fixed on something only she could perceive. Nothing had changed. The universe had reset.

I walked over to Louie, a quiet experiment playing out in my mind. "Louie," I began, my voice even, "did the Cubs win the World Series?"

Louie looked up, a familiar, contented expression on his face. "The Cubs won the World Series," he confirmed, as if it were the most natural, undeniable fact in the world. He then returned to his breakfast, his peace unbroken.

Mary, still at the window, turned her head slightly, her eyes distant but her voice clear. "Such a pretty song," she hummed, as if responding to an unheard melody.

In that moment, a quiet sense of understanding settled over me. The world outside might change, seasons might turn, but here, some truths were eternal, self-renewing with each dawn. Peace had been restored, for them, and in a strange way, for me too. This was their reality, and my job was to witness it, to understand it, and to help them navigate it, one World Series victory at a time.

# Phillip

The nature of reality is a multifaceted concept that intertwines philosophy, science, and personal experience. It challenges us to reconsider our assumptions about existence and encourages an ongoing exploration of what it means to be aware and to perceive the world around us. As we delve into these discussions, we recognize that reality may be as much about our interpretations and experiences as it is about the objective world itself. This philosophical lens, often a comfortable distance from the lived experience of suffering, became uncomfortably, starkly physical the day I met Phillip.

For Phillip, and countless others confined within the sprawling, echoing wards of Manteno State Hospital, the delicate architecture of reality had not merely shifted; it had fractured, splintered into a thousand agonizing pieces. My role there, as a caseworker, often felt like an exercise in mapping these shattered landscapes, trying to find a common ground, a shared coordinate between their world and ours. It was a thankless, often heartbreaking task, a daily confrontation with minds that had, for various, often inexplicable reasons, lost their mooring in what most of us consider "real."

Phillip, however, was different. His case, arriving on my desk amidst a stack of others — each a testament to a life derailed — presented not just a challenge to my professional capabilities, but a profound and unsettling interrogation of my own understanding of existence. He wasn't merely disconnected; he seemed to operate under a different set of rules entirely, rules that, in their own terrifying consistency, forced me to question whether my objective world was quite as objective as I comfortably believed.

His reality was not just an interpretation; it was a parallel universe, one I was compelled to navigate, often blindly, as I sought to understand the man behind the diagnoses. It was through Phillip's eyes, or rather, through the fragmented shards of his perception, that the abstract discussions of reality's fluidity ceased to be academic and became, instead, the very bedrock of a life, and my desperate attempt to touch it.

The chill of the Illinois winter had long settled into the bones of Manteno State Hospital, an old leviathan of brick and slate that swallowed lives whole. Phillip's arrival shattered whatever semblance of routine I had managed to construct. I still remember the rustle, almost like a dry leaf caught in a perpetual breeze, that preceded him down the corridor. When he finally stood before me, in the sterile, fluorescent glare of the admissions office, my breath hitched. Phillip was covered. Completely. From the crown of his head, where the silver gleamed under the strip lights, down to his heavily taped shoes, he was encased in a shimmering, crinkling suit of aluminum foil.

His eyes, wide and unnervingly lucid amidst the metallic sheen, met mine. There was no theatricality in his posture, no hint of a joke. He simply stood, a man in a human-sized, crinkled cocoon.

"My neighbor," he began, his voice surprisingly soft, almost apologetic, "he's sending the waves. Radio waves. Straight into my heart, Brian." He gestured vaguely towards his chest, the foil around his hand protesting with a whisper. "This... this is my protection. It bounces them right off."

My clipboard felt suddenly heavy in my hand. Manteno saw many things, dealt with countless iterations of fractured reality, but a man arriving head-to-toe in a self-fashioned suit of Reynolds Wrap was, even for us, a striking image. This wasn't just another file. This was Phillip, and his story—his battle against the invisible currents that assailed his heart—had just begun to unfold, right there in the admissions office, under the watchful, if slightly bewildered, gaze of his new caseworker.

Phillip was a man adrift, his reality tethered to a phantom threat – the omnipresent, insidious whisper of radio waves that he believed were being used to probe, to control, to steal his very thoughts and rupture his heart. It was a delusion, I knew, but it was his truth. And in its grip, he was a prisoner within the already imposing walls of Manteno.

His eyes, a startlingly clear blue against his gaunt face, held a perpetual wariness, an anxious darting that spoke of constant vigilance. He'd instinctively wrapped himself in layers of aluminum foil, a makeshift shield against an invisible enemy. But the foil, while offering him a semblance of protection, also served to further isolate him, to mark him as "other" in a place already teeming with the marginalized. I saw not just a patient, but a soul desperately clinging to some semblance of agency, albeit in a distorted form.

My immediate, overwhelming priority wasn't the sterile efficiency of psychiatric treatment charts or the prescribed protocols. It was the raw, vulnerable humanity I saw before me. How could I begin to help Phillip navigate the external world, let alone his internal one, when he was so fundamentally shielded, not just from imagined rays, but from connection, from trust, from his own inherent dignity? I knew, with a certainty that settled deep in my gut, that such a visible manifestation of his illness would make him a prime target for the casual cruelty that could fester in the undercurrents of any institution. Others, those who saw only a man in foil, would inevitably exploit his vulnerability.

So, faced with this immediate need, I improvised. It wasn't a textbook intervention; it was a spur-of-the-moment gambit born from a desperate desire to offer him a different perspective. Standing in the stark, echoing hallway, beside Phillip, I knocked firmly on the thick, unyielding concrete wall that lined the corridor. The thud reverberated, a solid, undeniable sound. "Phillip," I said, my voice deliberately pitched to be reassuring, yet firm, "these walls, they're built thick. Solid concrete. No radio waves can pierce these walls. You are safe here."

He turned his head, his blue eyes, sharp with suspicion, met mine. A flicker of uncertainty crossed his face, followed by a deep-seated anxiety. He wanted to believe me, I could see it in the slight softening of his posture, the way his gaze lingered on the wall as if trying to absorb its solidity. But for Phillip, my words weren't a simple reassurance; they were a suggested paradigm shift. I hadn't banished the radio waves, not truly. Instead, I had introduced a counter-narrative, a fragile seed of doubt planted in the fertile soil of his delusion. I had, for that brief, charged moment, suggested a shift in his reality, and the tentative hope warring with ingrained fear in his eyes was my only immediate gauge of its impact.

For several minutes I wondered if Phillip had heard too many stories, too many conspiracy theories. I realized that what was once thought of as a conspiracy theory was actually true. In 1932, the U.S. Public Health Service, working with the Tuskegee Institute, began a study to record the natural history of syphilis. It was originally called the "Tuskegee Study of Untreated Syphilis in the Negro Male" (now referred to as the "USPHS Untreated Syphilis Study at Tuskegee"). The study initially involved 600 Black men – 399 with syphilis, 201 who did not have the disease. Participants' informed consent was not collected. Researchers told the men they were being treated for "bad blood," a local term used to describe several ailments, including syphilis, anemia, and fatigue. In exchange for taking part in the study, the men received free medical exams, free meals, and burial insurance.

The thoughts blurred my mind, but the implications sharpened into a terrible clarity. My stomach clenched. For years, I, like many others, had dismissed the wilder claims of patients here at Manteno as symptoms of their illness, the flotsam of a broken mind. "They're experimenting on us," someone might whisper, or "They tell us one thing, but they're doing another." We had our protocols, our diagnoses, our neatly categorized delusions. But what if those delusions were, at their origin, not delusions at all? What if they were the distorted echoes of real, profound betrayals?

Phillip, with his perpetually nervous gaze and his habit of clutching his threadbare blanket even in the summer heat, had often spoken of feeling like a "guinea pig." He'd never been coherent enough to articulate his fears with precision, often circling back to vague notions of people "messing with his head." I'd recorded it in his file as paranoid ideation, a classic manifestation of his schizophrenia, perhaps exacerbated by the institutional setting. Now, the phrase "bad blood" from the Tuskegee report echoed in my ears, a chilling parallel to Phillip's own fragmented anxieties.

The weight of my own prior dismissal settled heavily on me. How many times had I nodded empathetically, while internally cataloging another instance of a patient's disconnect from reality? How many times had I assured a frightened man or woman that they were safe, that we were here to help, while a part of me subconsciously believed their fears were unfounded fantasies?

During that time Manteno was a sprawling, often understaffed facility. We prided ourselves on what we could do, the therapies we offered, the semblance of order we maintained. But beneath that veneer, there was always the quiet hum of patient discontent, a low thrum of suspicion that I now understood came from a far deeper, far more ancient source than mere mental illness. It was a suspicion rooted in history, in the knowledge—passed down through whispers, through unspoken cultural memory—that institutions, even those meant to heal, could inflict unimaginable harm.

My next meeting with Phillip was scheduled for later that afternoon. I looked at my notes, at the clinical language I'd used to describe his "paranoid tendencies," and felt a profound shame. I wasn't just a caseworker anymore; I was a man now burdened by a horrifying truth. My approach to Phillip, and to every patient in my care, had to change. I had to listen not just for the symptoms, but for the echoes of history, for the buried truths that might be masquerading as madness. Phillip wasn't just my patient; he was a gatekeeper to a grim understanding, and I had finally begun to listen.

Phillip's fingers, thin and pale, tightened around the glass. His knuckles glowed white against the transparent surface, a stark contrast to the vivid, imagined terrors within. His gaze was fixed, not on the water itself, but on something just beneath its surface, something only visible through the unique lens of his mind.

"They're... busy today," he murmured, his voice a dry whisper that seemed to scratch against the quiet hum of Manteno. "The reds are particularly agitated. Always the angriest, those ones. And the blue... the blue is watching, waiting for the red to do its worst." He tilted the glass slightly, as if examining a rare specimen. A shiver ran through his gaunt frame. "The green, though," he added, his eyes meeting mine briefly, a flash of profound, weary fear. "The green is the cleverest. It tricks you. Hides."

I kept my expression neutral, resisting the urge to offer a logical counter-argument. Logic, I had learned, was a language Phillip no longer fully understood, or rather, it was a language spoken in a different dialect from his own. "It's just fresh water, Phillip," I said softly, my voice calm and even. "From the tap. It's safe."

He recoiled slightly at my words, as if they were a foreign, disturbing sound. Slowly, deliberately, he placed the glass back on the small, chipped bedside table. His eyes, faded and distant, returned to me, carrying an almost pitying look. "You can't see them, can you, Brian?" he asked, his voice softer now, tinged with a strange, sorrowful knowing. The water sat untouched, a silent, shimmering barrier between two realities.

I left Phillip's room that day with my clipboard untouched, the water still glinting on the bedside table. I didn't chart his words. I didn't correct his colors. I simply carried them with me—red, blue, green—like coordinates from a map I hadn't learned to read. And maybe that's what it means to bear witness: not to fix, not to explain, but to stand quietly beside a man who sees what you cannot, and to let his vision alter your own.

The institutional linoleum groaned under my worn shoes as I walked away, the fluorescent hum of the ward replacing the soft murmur of Phillip's voice. He had been tracing patterns in the air, his fingers alight with an unseen energy. "Red," he'd said, pointing to the corner of the ceiling where a shadow usually lay, "that's where the fear collects, Brian. It's a heavy, pulsing red, like a drum beating too fast." Then, his gaze shifted to the window, to the bare branch scratching against the pane. "But the hope," he'd whispered, a rare, almost shy smile touching his lips, "the hope is a faint blue, like the underside of a sparrow's wing. It tries to get out, always. And you, Brian," he'd fixed me with those startlingly clear eyes, "you carry a steady green today. Like a deep root. It settles the red."

My training, the endless hours of lectures on diagnostic criteria and therapeutic interventions, had equipped me with tools to categorize Phillip, to label his experiences as symptoms of a fractured mind. My colleagues, seasoned by years of Manteno's relentless rhythm, would have scribbled "hallucinations" or "delusional ideation" without a second thought, perhaps prescribing a stronger sedative. But Phillip's green, the steady root he'd seen in me, felt more real than any official diagnosis. It was a warmth I hadn't realized I needed, a confirmation that I wasn't just a cog in this colossal, often dehumanizing machine.

The scent of antiseptic and stale coffee clung to the air, a constant reminder of where I was. Other patients shuffled in the dayroom, some lost in their own internal landscapes, others staring blankly at the flickering television. Each face held a story, but Manteno's purpose was to manage, not always to listen. It was a place designed to contain the chaotic, to smooth the jagged edges of human suffering into something more palatable for society, even if it meant dulling the very essence of a person.

I found myself leaning against a cold concrete wall, the clipboard a dead weight in my hand. What good would it do to write "Patient reports seeing colors associated with emotions"? It would be filed, dismissed, maybe even used to justify another increase in his medication. It would deny the validity of his experience, stamp it as pathology. And what if his pathology was a different way of seeing the world, a heightened sensitivity to truths I was too numb, too conditioned to perceive?

My initial purpose at Manteno had been clear: to assess, to document, to facilitate whatever small improvements were possible within the rigid framework of the institution. But with Phillip, the lines blurred. He wasn't just a patient; he was a teacher, albeit an unwitting one, peeling back layers of my own professional detachment. He was forcing me to confront the limitations of my understanding, to question the very definition of sanity.

I thought of the water on his bedside table, still and clear, reflecting the harsh light. He hadn't touched it, preferring instead to navigate his internal currents. And I hadn't touched my clipboard, because some truths, some visions, were too profound to be reduced to ink on a page. They needed to be carried, felt, allowed to infuse the very way you saw the world.

As I turned down the long, echoing corridor towards my office, I knew my visits with Phillip would no longer be about charting his illness, but about learning to read the colors he painted on the canvas of our shared, bewildering reality.

I used to think delusions were distortions—misfires of the mind, symptoms to be managed. But Phillip taught me that some delusions are not delusions at all. They are echoes. Inherited truths too jagged for protocol. And if we listen closely, not with charts but with mercy, we might hear in their cadence the history we've tried to forget. The foil, the colors, the water—they weren't madness. They were memory.

Phillip didn't ask to be understood. He asked to be remembered. And I, the caseworker, finally stopped managing and started listening. Not to symptoms, but to echoes. Not to madness, but to memory. The foil shimmered. The colors pulsed. And the water, untouched, reflected a truth too jagged for protocol.

# Jerry

Jerry walked slowly. He talked slowly. He never said much unless he was spoken to. He couldn't hold a conversation. He had come to Manteno after a bout with phencyclidine (PCP) commonly known on the street as "angel dust." PCP is a dissociative drug that can cause hallucinations, distorted perceptions, and severe psychological effects. PCP is a dissociative anesthetic that was originally developed in the 1950s for use as an intravenous anesthetic. Due to severe side effects, including hallucinations and agitation, its medical use was discontinued. PCP is considered one of the more dangerous drugs due to its potential for addiction and severe psychological effects. Regular use can lead to psychological dependence and cravings. High doses can result in violent behavior, paranoia, and severe mood swings. Overdose can lead to seizures, coma, and even death. Long-term use may result in lasting cognitive impairments and mental health issues.

Jerry's quiet, shuffling form was a constant, stark reminder of the battles being fought within these walls. He wasn't on my official caseload, but it was impossible to work at Manteno and not notice Jerry. He was one of the many spectral figures who haunted the sun-bleached common rooms and sterile hallways, a living monument to the destructive power of a single chemical compound.

I'd often see him in the day room, perched on the edge of an armchair, staring at a television that wasn't on, his eyes wide and vacant. Sometimes, he'd slowly turn his head, his gaze sweeping across the room as if searching for something just beyond the periphery of his sight.

There was a profound stillness to Jerry that spoke volumes. It wasn't peace; it was the quiet of a mind that had been violently disrupted, its connections frayed, its natural rhythms silenced. The doctors had noted his condition as a persistent post-PCP psychosis, a lingering shadow that had refused to lift after his initial acute episode. He was in his mid-thirties, but the drug had aged him, etching lines of worry and confusion onto a face that should have been unblemished. More than that, PCP is stored in the fat cells of the body. A change in weight could re-activate the effects of PCP. His slow walk had a purpose. Jerry's slow walk wasn't just a symptom—it was choreography. A ritual of containment. A sovereign adaptation to a body that could betray him at any moment.

I'd walk past him during sessions, or see him during meal times, meticulously pushing food around his plate, sometimes taking a bite, sometimes just letting it sit. I remember one afternoon, I knelt beside him, trying to engage, offering a gentle "Hello, Jerry. How are you today?" His eyes, deep brown and clouded, slowly met mine. A flicker of something – fear? recognition? – crossed them, then vanished.

He offered no verbal response, only a faint, almost imperceptible nod, before his gaze drifted back to the empty television screen. It was a small interaction, but it left a profound impression. It hammered home the quiet despair that permeated Manteno, the silent suffering of individuals whose very ability to connect with the world had been fractured. Jerry was a living testament to the silent, enduring damage that a moment of altered perception could inflict, consigning a man to a life lived in the twilight of his own mind. He wasn't just a casualty of PCP. He was a living footnote to the pharmacological optimism of the 1950s, the institutional choreography of containment, and the ensemble grief of those who bore witness.

But one day, Jerry walked to the pool table, racked the balls, and issued a loud crack as the pool balls scurried about the table. He proceeded to run the table. Then, he did it again. This time he displayed his mastery of the game, hitting triple bank shots, double bank shots, impossible shots. And yet, he never once celebrated a shot or showed any enthusiasm for the game.

I had been in the corner, idly flipping through a patient file, a small defense against the pervasive dullness that often settled upon the Manteno recreation room. But the sharp, successive clicks of balls finding their pockets, followed by the stunned silence from the usual boisterous group around the table, pulled my attention away from the dry prose. My gaze landed on Jerry, who had, until this moment, been a study in quiet inertia. He was a man carved from institutional routine, a fixture in his chosen chair by the window, staring out at nothing in particular. He barely spoke, rarely initiated interaction, and never, in my experience, displayed any discernible interest in the world beyond the immediate reach of his vacant stare.

And then—Jerry cracked the silence.

Not with words, not with a speech, but with geometry. With precision. With a sovereign choreography of angles and force that defied every assumption Manteno had made about him. That pool table wasn't recreation—it was revelation. A ritual of memory, maybe muscle, maybe myth. Triple bank shots, impossible shots—each one a dispatch from a part of Jerry that hadn't been erased, only buried. And when he ran the table again, without celebration, without even a flicker of pride, it wasn't detachment. It was editorial restraint. A refusal to perform joy for an audience that had already written him off

Jerry simply stood there, cue held loosely, like an artist who had just completed a masterpiece but felt no connection to the work. There was no triumphant grin, no subtle nod of satisfaction, no spark in his eyes. He merely surveyed the table, the balls now perfectly arranged in their pockets, and then, as if the entire performance had been nothing more than a momentary glitch in the predictable rhythm of his existence, he placed the cue in its rack.

Without a backward glance, without acknowledging the stunned silence or the wide-eyed stares directed his way, Jerry walked away from the pool table. He moved with the same slow, deliberate gait he always had, and without hesitation, resumed his usual spot by the radiator, his gaze once again fixed on a chip in the peeling paint. It was as if some other entity had taken momentary possession of his body, a ghost of a forgotten life peeking through the fog of his illness, only to retreat just as quickly.

I felt a surge of something I hadn't felt in a long time with Jerry: not exactly hope, but a profound, unsettling curiosity. For weeks, months even, he had been a cipher, a patient whose case file offered little, and whose presence offered less. But in those brief, stunning minutes, he had revealed a hidden depth, a dormant brilliance that defied everything I thought I knew about him.

It was a stark reminder that even within the confines of Manteno, beneath the layers of diagnosis and institutional routine, there were still vast, unexplored territories of the human spirit.

Clearly, the staff saw an opportunity to showcase Jerry's talent. We organized a hospital-wide pool tournament. Opponent after opponent merely watched as Jerry dropped ball after ball. When he was finished, he'd ask, "Can I go now?" Bets were made. Our unit had a secret weapon. He not only won every game, but he also never missed a shot!

This wasn't the Jerry I'd come to know over the past months at Manteno State Hospital. The Jerry who had sat with me while sitting on the unit, his gaze drifting towards the barred windows, his words hesitant and often trailing off into silence. The Jerry who struggled to engage, who flinched at sudden movements, who seemed lost in a fog I couldn't penetrate. This was a different Jerry. This was a Jerry who commanded attention, his hands steady as they chalked the cue, his eyes sharp and focused on the table.

The pool tournament was the brainchild of recreation therapist, a man who possessed an uncanny ability to see beyond the diagnosis, to ferret out the sparks of humanity that flickered within each patient. He had noticed Jerry's quiet fascination with the battered pool table in the recreation room, the way his eyes would follow the trajectory of the balls, the subtle tension in his shoulders when others played. "He's got a touch, Brian," he had confided in me, his voice a low hum of conviction. "A real touch."

And he was right. What unfolded that afternoon defied expectations, defying the somber reality of Manteno. In the hushed anticipation of the crowd, Jerry was transformed. The hesitant, withdrawn man I knew evaporated, replaced by a confident artist of the felt. His movements were fluid, precise. The crack of the cue ball was the only sound that punctuated the gallery's stunned silence. Each shot was a masterpiece, a testament to an innate skill that had lain dormant, unseen.

When the final ball sank, the room erupted in a mixture of cheers and bewildered applause. Jerry, his face impassive, looked at me, a question in his eyes, a relic of his usual demeanor. "Can I go now?" he asked, the words a familiar refrain.

He had shown us more than just his skill at pool; he had shown us a glimpse of the man buried beneath the illness, a man capable of precision, of focus, of winning. And in that moment, standing there amidst the lingering echo of the last shot, I felt a surge of hope, a quiet understanding that my work with Jerry was about to become far more complex, and far more rewarding, than I had ever imagined.

The silence that descended was heavier than any I'd experienced in Jerry's presence. It wasn't just the disappointment of the missed shot, though that hung thick and cloying in the air. It was the palpable deflation of Jerry himself, a man who, for all his fractured realities and admitted delusions, had found a sliver of genuine triumph in this sterile, fluorescent-lit recreation room.

I watched. Jerry's shoulders didn't slump. The usual spark in his eyes, the one that flickered to life when he talked about his intricate theories or his plans for a world beyond Manteno's walls, remained. He stood frozen for a moment, the cue stick still in his hand, a question mark etched onto his face. The supposed "easy shot" had not become his undoing, not by any physical failing on his part, but by the insidious, whispered suggestion that preyed on his deepest insecurities.

The other staff members, moments before beaming with pride at their patient's prowess, now shifted uncomfortably. Some offered half-hearted murmurs of "Almost, Jerry," or "Tough break." But their words felt hollow, mere platitudes to fill the void left by Jerry's failure. The forensic patient, a hulking shadow named Marcus whose quiet demeanor usually masked a sharp intellect, offered no further comment. He simply returned to his seat, a faint, unreadable smile playing on his lips.

I walked over to Jerry, the worn linoleum floor squeaking faintly under my shoes. He didn't look at me, his gaze fixed on the billiard table, on the mocking white of the eight ball sitting innocently in its pocket. I knew this routine. I'd seen it play out in countless smaller arenas within Manteno – in games of chess, in debates about current events, even in the simple act of sharing a meal. Jerry could build empires in his mind, could outwit imaginary adversaries with dazzling logic, but the faintest tremor of doubt, amplified by external suggestion, could crumble his carefully constructed realities.

"Hey, Jerry," I said softly, my voice cutting through the heavy quiet. I didn't address the missed shot directly. Instead, I gestured towards the table. "Good game. You really had him on the ropes."

He finally turned to me, his face a mask of weary resignation. His hands, which had been steady as he lined up the shot, now trembled slightly. He ran a hand through his thinning hair, a nervous habit I recognized all too well.

"He shouldn't have said that, Brian," Jerry finally managed, his voice raspy.

And there it was. The core of it. Not the missed shot, not the championship title, but the knowledge that someone else, another patient in this very institution, had understood his vulnerability and exploited it. It was a betrayal, not of sportsmanship, but of the fragile trust that sometimes bloomed in the most unlikely of places. It was a stark reminder of the delicate balance Jerry, and so many others here, maintained, and how easily it could be tipped. The imagined purchases, the gloating staff, the championship – all of it had dissolved into the same bitter air. Now, all that remained was the raw, exposed nerve of Jerry's Achilles' heel, and the quiet, lingering question of what would happen next.

True to form, nothing happened next. Jerry still walked slowly. Jerry still talked slowly. Jerry was Jerry, still running the table. He had the skill, but not the ego. And, in its way, we wondered if, in an attempt to elevate this man, we truly exploited him.

The billiard room, a dimly lit sanctuary within the sprawling, often sterile halls of Manteno State Hospital, had become Jerry's domain. It was the one place where his internal world, so often a labyrinth of fragmented thoughts and gentle confusion, found a clear path. The click of the balls, the smooth slide of the cue, the satisfying thud as they settled into pockets – these were the rhythms that anchored him.

He'd arrive each afternoon, a worn wooden cue stick held with careful reverence, his gaze already fixed on the green felt as if it held the secrets of the universe. He'd line up shots with an uncanny precision, a silent ballet of physics and intuition that few of us, his supposed caregivers, could comprehend.

My role, as his caseworker, was to observe, to document, to facilitate. It sounded so clinical, so detached. But spending hours in that room, watching Jerry navigate the geometric challenges of the game, chipped away at the professional distance. It was hard not to get invested. He wasn't just a case file; he was the man who could sink a seven-ball on the break with startling regularity, who would smile a slow, genuine smile when he pulled off a particularly tricky bank shot. He was the man who, when I'd finally gather the courage to ask about his life before Manteno, would offer fragments: a mention of a factory job, a sister's wedding, the taste of a good cup of coffee. These were precious, ephemeral glimpses into a life that had been so drastically altered, so profoundly misunderstood by the world outside.

And so, the question lingered – was this "elevation" of Jerry, this focus on his undeniable talent, a genuine step towards recognizing his personhood, or was it a way for us, the staff, to feel we were doing something meaningful with a patient who might otherwise be overlooked? Was his skill a genuine source of pride and agency for him, or was it a performance, a carefully curated act that masked a deeper despair?

As I watched him meticulously rack the balls after another victory, his expression unchanged, the weight of that ethical quandary pressed down on me, heavy as a loaded cue ball. Had we found a way to bring Jerry out of himself, or had we simply found a way to make ourselves feel better about keeping him here?

And so, the question lingered – was this "elevation" of Jerry, this focus on his undeniable talent, a genuine step towards recognizing his personhood, or was it a way for us, the staff, to feel we were doing something meaningful with a patient who might otherwise be overlooked? Was his skill a genuine source of pride and agency for him, or was it a performance, a carefully curated act that masked a deeper despair?

As I watched him meticulously rack the balls after another victory, his expression unchanged, the weight of that ethical quandary pressed down on me, heavy as a loaded cue ball. Had we found a way to bring Jerry out of himself, or had we simply found a way to make ourselves feel better about keeping him here?

# Bill

The fluorescent lights of Manteno State Hospital hummed a low, constant drone, a lullaby of sorts for the souls held within its walls. It was a sound I'd become accustomed to, a backdrop to the quiet desperation and the occasional outbursts that punctuated daily life. When I arrived, the name Bill was already etched into the hospital's history, a ghost from a time I hadn't yet witnessed.

Bill had walked through these doors twenty years before me. Twenty years. The words themselves felt heavy, weighted with the passage of time and the stillness of a life arrested. He'd entered not as a criminal, but as a man deemed incapable of understanding the weight of his own actions. The court, in its pronouncement, had uttered the letters NGRI – Not Guilty by Reason of Insanity. His severe paranoid schizophrenia, a fierce storm raging within his mind, had rendered him a stranger to justice, a victim of his own fractured reality.

The verdict wasn't a key to freedom, not in the way the world outside understood it. Instead, it was a passage, a solemn transfer from the iron bars of criminal justice to the more subtle, yet equally confining, walls of the mental health system. It was a declaration not of innocence, but of incapacity. The law, in its intricate dance, stepped back, recognizing that punishment was a futile endeavor for a mind that couldn't grasp the wrongfulness of its own deeds, a mind lost in the labyrinth of its delusions.

For Manteno, and for Bill, this meant a life dedicated to treatment, to the slow, arduous process of managing a condition that offered no easy cure. It meant a different kind of sentence, measured not in years but in the ebb and flow of his symptoms, in the quiet mornings and the restless nights, under the watchful eyes of those dedicated to his care. He was a man whose story began not with conviction, but with an acknowledgment of a profound internal battle, a battle that had landed him here, twenty years before I ever knew his name. And as I learned more about Bill, I realized his story wasn't just about his past offense, but about the long, complex journey of living with a mind that played by different rules, in a world that struggled to understand.

The sterile scent of disinfectant was the first thing Bill registered, a familiar, unwelcome perfume that clung to the institutional air. Sunlight, filtered through the barred windows of the common dayroom, painted stripes across the worn linoleum floor. Bill traced one of these stripes with the toe of his sensible, government-issue slipper. He was in his third year at Chester – a facility for the criminally insane—a place he'd been sent by a judge's gavel rather than a jury's verdict. Not guilty by reason of insanity – NGRI. The words still felt foreign, a label that had been slapped onto him, defining him by a moment of profound darkness he barely remembered.

The commitment wasn't a prison sentence, at least not in the traditional sense. There were no set dates, no ticking clock towards freedom. Instead, it was an open-ended mandate: stay here, get better, prove you're no longer a danger. The 'danger' part, Bill knew, was the highest hurdle, a mountain of anxiety and delusion he'd been painstakingly chipping away at, one therapy session, one medication adjustment, one quiet evening at a time.

His days were structured. Mornings were for group therapy, where the raw edges of fractured minds were sometimes smoothed, sometimes snagged on each other like barbed wire. Afternoons were for individual sessions with his psychologist, a man with kind eyes and a voice that could soothe or probe with equal precision, yet still conflicted. Bill was guilty of a heinous crime.

Bill had embraced the regimen. He took his meds religiously, even when the side effects made him feel like a stranger in his own skin.

He attended every group, spoke when he felt he could, and listened intently when he couldn't. He'd learned the names of his fellow patients, their stories whispered over lukewarm coffee, each a testament to the fragility of the human psyche. There was Sarah, who saw constellations in the ceiling tiles, and Mark, who believed he was a chess grandmaster playing against an invisible opponent. Bill, in his own way, had found a quiet corner of stability within the storm.

The annual reviews were the nerve-wracking punctuation marks in his otherwise monotonous year. The treatment team, a collection of doctors, nurses, and therapists, would gather. They'd pore over his progress reports, his engagement levels, his reported insights. Bill would sit, his breath shallow, his heart a frantic drum against his ribs, waiting for their assessment. He knew the legal standard was "clear and convincing evidence." Not just a hint of improvement, but a solid, undeniable demonstration that the illness that had once consumed him was now a manageable shadow, not a rampaging beast.

His first review had been a disaster. He'd been too anxious, too eager to please, his words tumbling out in a frantic rush. They'd seen his fear, not his progress. The second review had been better. He'd managed to articulate his understanding of his illness, his triggers, his coping mechanisms. But still, the decision had been to continue commitment. The fear, a residual echo, had been enough.

This year felt different. He'd had a breakthrough in his individual therapy. His psychologist had helped him unpack the tangled mess of guilt and confusion that had surrounded the incident. He could finally look at himself in the mirror, not as a monster, but as a man who had been severely ill and was now on a path to recovery.

The day of the review arrived like any other, the sun rising, the birds chirping their indifferent songs outside. Bill dressed carefully, his hands steady. He walked into the conference room, the air thick with the usual sterile scent, but for Bill, it also smelled faintly of hope. He sat, composed, and met the gaze of each team member. He spoke not of what he hoped for, but of what he knew. He described his understanding of his illness with a clarity that surprised even himself. He spoke of the strategies he employed to manage his anxieties, the support system he was building, even within the confines of the hospital.

He watched their faces, searching for subtle shifts. He saw nods of acknowledgement, thoughtful frowns, and then, finally, a small smile from his psychologist, a man who determined that the best way to gauge Bill's readiness for release was to measure whether or not Bill had felt any remorse for his crimes. And so, Bill was asked to recall the events of that day twenty years earlier while we watched and listened.

The silence in the room was thick, heavy with the unspoken weight of twenty years. Bill's voice, once a vibrant tenor, now rasped, each word a shard of glass scraped from a broken past. He stared at his hands, gnarled and weathered, as if they held the phantom weight of a child.

"Twenty years ago," he began, his voice a low rumble, "I was married. Young. Thought I was well. I had a job, a life. Then... poof. Gone. Don't even remember why I lost it. Just... home. With the baby."

He paused, licking his dry lips. The memory, raw and festering, bled into the present. "My wife worked. So I was... the man of the house. Daycare provider. Couldn't stand it. The baby. Helpless. And me? Even more so. The crying..." His voice cracked. "That damn crying. It was a constant buzz, a high-pitched needle in my brain. Sometimes I'd just... leave it. Let it wail itself out. Sometimes I'd rock it. Nothing. Nothing ever stopped the crying."

A shiver traced its way down his spine. "She'd come home," he continued, his gaze unfocused, "and find me outside. Shade myself from the sun while the baby screamed its lungs out inside. She'd yell. I'd promise. 'Never again, I swear.' Lies. All lies. I was sick. So damn sick. She... she didn't know. But I did. I was a father who hated his own child."

He squeezed his eyes shut, as if to block out the spectral image. "Then, the next morning," he whispered, the words barely audible, "before she left... she told me. She told me... I wasn't the daddy. Some other man. Not me. And the baby... it was crying again. While she... she left. Went to him, I guess. Or work. I don't know. Never knew where she went. She just... vanished. And I was stuck. With the baby. Not mine. And it was crying."

His breath hitched. "I picked it up. Looked at its face. Crying. Always crying. And something snapped. The anger... it just boiled over. 'You're not my baby,' I thought. 'You're not mine.' I was tricked. Fooled. And now she's gone, and I'm here with this... this thing. Crying. And I... I hated it."

He leaned forward, his forearms resting on his knees, his hands clasped so tightly his knuckles were white. "Twenty years," he repeated, the words a broken melody. "Twenty years I've replayed it. That baby. The one I picked up... and smashed. To the floor." His voice dropped to a guttural growl. "I remember it. Still see it. On the floor. Not my baby. Someone else's. I... I killed it."

The confession hung in the air, a brutal, undeniable truth. Tears, hot and thick, finally spilled down his weathered cheeks, carving streaks through the dirt and the years of pain. "I didn't mean to," he choked out, his body wracked by silent sobs. "But I did. God forgive me, but I did. I still see it... where I sat. Rocking. Crying."

After he finished speaking, he was asked to leave the room while we debated that what we had heard from Bill was remorse—enough to recommend his release. He was called back after thirty minutes of discussion. He walked in fully expecting we would decline his release. But we announced we would recommend his release to a supervised halfway home. After which, Bill still need to follow the court ordered supervision.

The review was over. The papers were signed. The recommendation made. Bill had left the room, his slippers quiet against the linoleum. But long after he was gone, the silence remained. The chair he'd occupied still faced us, slightly askew. And in that silence, we wondered—not whether Bill was ready, but whether we were. If remorse is enough to release a man, is it ever enough to release the memory?

# The Naked Runner

Manteno was not an urban monolith, but rather an institution deeply embedded in the quiet, expansive embrace of the American heartland. It sat, isolated and imposing, deep in the country, its manicured but stark grounds giving way almost immediately to the rhythm of agricultural life. Beyond its fences, beyond its last neatly trimmed hedge, stretched an unbroken quilt of farmland. And on that farmland, dominating the horizon, were acres upon acres of corn.

This verdant expanse, beautiful in its own stark, rural way, served a practical, if unintentional, purpose. It was a natural barrier. For anyone inside the facility who might consider leaving the hospital grounds without authorization, the cornfield presented a formidable, often disorienting, challenge. These individuals were known, with a stark simplicity, as "runners."

"Runners" was a term used as shorthand for those who, for reasons we could not always ascertain – a sudden impulse, a profound delusion, a desperate longing for freedom – would simply decide to run away from the facility. It was a common issue, a recurring phenomenon that spoke to the complex inner worlds of Manteno's residents. And it was potentially harmful. The cornfield, with its towering stalks that could quickly swallow a person whole, its labyrinthine paths, and the sheer, disorienting expanse of it, posed a significant threat to anyone who ventured into its depths without proper guidance or preparation. Disorientation, exposure to the elements, injury, or simply being lost—these were not uncommon fates for those who sought refuge or escape within its whispering walls.

On one particular day, the name of which is lost to the passage of time, as is her own, a woman became one of those runners. We recall her not by identity, but by action. Perhaps it was a flicker of sunlight through a window that called to her, a distant sound carried on the wind, or an internal whisper that no one else could hear. Whatever the catalyst, the decision was made, silently, profoundly.

She seized an opportunity, a moment of unguarded passage, and moved. Not with stealth, perhaps, but with a sudden, unleashed energy that propelled her forward. Her steps, at first hurried across the closer, flatter earth, soon found purchase on the softer, tilled soil bordering the fields. And then, she was there. At the edge of the towering stalks, which at that time of year, could easily eclipse a person, standing several feet taller than the average man.

Without hesitation, or perhaps with a surge of desperate resolve, she plunged into the dense green. The rustling leaves closed in around her, the air grew heavy and still, and the outside world—the facility she had just fled—vanished from view. She became a moving shadow within the endless rows, another whisper among the rustling stalks. A runner, lost to the corn, and for a crucial period, to the immediate knowledge of those who remained behind. Her reasons, like those of so many runners, remained her own, buried somewhere in the vast, silent expanse she had chosen to embrace, however briefly, as her escape.

The first time I saw her, I thought it was a mirage. The summer heat shimmered off the asphalt of the service road, distorting the world, and then this figure emerged from the side door of Building B – a discreet exit, usually kept locked, or at least meticulously monitored. She wasn't a patient from my unit; I worked in a different unit. But her name, or rather, the idea of her, was a common currency among staff hospital-wide. A whispered warning exchanged during shift reports.

"Keep an eye out for her, especially if you're near the north end," someone would often say, their voices tinged with a blend of exasperation and a strange, almost grudging respect. "She's known to bolt."

And bolt she did.

What made her unique, what truly cemented her legend in the annals of this sprawling, brick-and-mortar facility, was her chosen attire for these escapes. Or, rather, her decided lack of it. Not a stitch of clothing. Ever.

I never understood it. How did she find the moment? Was it a sudden, primal urge that overcame her, shedding constraints both mental and physical in one swift, furious movement? Did she meticulously plan, folding her clothing into a neat pile before bursting forth, or were they ripped away in a frenzy of pure instinct? The sheer logistics of it always baffled me. I never observed the prelude, never witnessed that pivotal moment where a patient transformed into a streaking, unburdened enigma.

My sightings, like everyone else's, always began mid-stride.

That first time, the afternoon sun glinted off her pale skin as she sprinted across the dry grass, a surprisingly graceful, almost ethereal blur against the stark green of the fields. Her arms pumped, her head was thrown back, and her hair, dark and unbound, streamed behind her like a banner. She was fast. Faster than she had any right to be, given the sedatives and structured routines that defined our world here.

Her target was always the same: the cornfield. A vast, rustling ocean of green stalks that bordered the hospital grounds, offering both concealment and, for a brief, glorious moment, a taste of unbound freedom. The staff would be right behind her, of course. A flurry of security guards, of orderlies, their walkie-talkies crackling with urgency, their faces grim as they pursued the most peculiar kind of escapee.

But for those few seconds, before the chase truly caught up, she was magnificent. A wild, uninhibited force of nature, propelled by some furious, inarticulate desire to be free of everything – the walls, the rules, the very clothes on her back. A naked woman, flying towards the cornfield, an unforgettable streak of defiance against the sterile backdrop of institutional life. And in those moments, you couldn't help but wonder what she was running towards, or more profoundly, what she was running from, with such desperate, beautiful abandon.

The sun beat down, turning the air between the towering stalks into a humid, oppressive soup. Each step was a commitment, pushing through the dense growth, the dry leaves scratching at our arms and faces. The rhythmic swish-swish of twenty pairs of legs moving through the corn was punctuated by an erratic, faster thrashing ahead of us – her.

"She's moving fast!" someone yelled, the voice muffled by the rustling. Ed grunted from a few paces to my left, his face already red and glistening with sweat. "Keep the line! Don't break formation!"

It was like trying to navigate a living maze, each row identical to the last, the sun a hazy glow above. We could hear her ragged breaths, the frantic beat of her bare feet on the soil, sometimes a low sob or a desperate whimper. She was terrified, but her fear fueled her, giving her a desperate strength. We, on the other hand, were just doing our jobs, our movements heavy with obligation and the growing discomfort of the heat and the constant, abrasive touch of the corn.

"My crops! You're crushing them!" The farmer's enraged bellow cut through the cacophony, a distant, furious counterpoint to our relentless advance. He was somewhere on the perimeter, running along the edge, his cries of agricultural anguish a familiar soundtrack to these unfortunate escapes. We tried to ignore him, but his words hung in the air, an added layer of guilt to an already thankless task.

The scent of dry earth and cut leaves filled my nostrils. My throat was dry. We'd been in there for what felt like an hour, pushing deeper, the field seemingly endless. Then, the thrashing ahead of us intensified, becoming more desperate, less a flight and more a frantic, cornered struggle. The sounds she made were no longer whimpers but sharp, guttural cries. We were closing in. The line tightened, each person quickening their pace, the unspoken urgency passing between us. The corn stalks, once an irritating barrier, now felt like prison bars, about to give way.

The heavy metal door of her unit clanged shut, a dull thud that always felt too final. The staff nurse, a weary woman named Brenda with tired eyes, simply nodded, taking the bundled Ed's jacket from the woman's shoulders as if it were a routine transaction. No questions, no thanks, just the silent acknowledgment of a situation resolved. Ed's "choice words" had been delivered in a low rumble, a frustrated grumble about vigilance and protocol, but Brenda had heard it all before. Her job was to keep them, not to chase them.

As for us, the giggling persisted, a quiet, almost conspiratorial sound as we walked back to the security vehicle. It wasn't just relief; it was the sheer, baffling humanity of it all. Who escapes into a cornfield just to sit and hum a little tune? It defied every expectation of panic, fear, or even a desperate plea. It wasn't an escape from something, but an escape to something – a brief, strange communion with rustling stalks and a private melody.

"You think she does that often?" I asked Ed, still chuckling as he started the engine. The field of broken cornstalks was visible in the rearview mirror, a jagged scar on the horizon.

Ed grunted, pulling out of the gravel drive. "Probably. They all got their quirks. Hers just happens to involve a pastoral interlude and a lot of damaged produce." He shook his head, a wry smile playing on his lips. "Bet the farmer's gonna love our incident report. 'Pursuit of resident led to extensive crop damage.'"

The walk back was filled with a comfortable silence, punctuated by the occasional shared look and a lingering chuckle. We were back to the mundane, the paperwork waiting, the next call inevitably coming. But for a few moments, the absurdity of the cornfield escape had momentarily lifted the usual weight of our work. It wasn't about the broken rules or the potential danger; it was about the unexpected, the utterly whimsical defiance of a woman who just wanted to hum in the corn.

That night, filling out the report, I found myself hesitating at the section marked 'Resident Behavior During Incident.' "Uncooperative?" No, not really. "Distressed?" Hardly. I finally wrote, "Found humming quietly, appeared calm and unbothered." It felt like an inadequate description for such a singular, peculiar moment, but it was the truth. And it reminded me, even in this job of rules and procedures, that sometimes, the most profound thing you could witness was a moment of unexpected, serene, and utterly unreasoned joy. Even if it did involve a cornfield and a very confused farmer.

Within a couple of weeks of that incident, some organization thought it would be nice to set up a small, not small, minimal carnival of sorts. Hardly a carnival. One ride. Food. Games. All patients were welcome, but few did more than eat. Let's be honest: they were adults, and the idea of a merry-go-round was off their radar.

Except hers.

We saw her striding towards us from a distance. The closer she got, the more naked she became.

She wasn't stripping in a frenzy, or as a display of distress. Each garment was removed with a deliberate, almost ritualistic precision. The shapeless hospital gown, the coarse undergarments, the socks—each was shed with a practiced movement, dropped onto the grass with no backward glance. By the time she reached the perimeter of the makeshift carnival, where the faint, tinny music of the sole ride was just audible, she was entirely nude. Her body, pale and stark, was perfectly unadorned, a living sculpture of determination.

Her eyes were fixed on the merry-go-round, not with the innocent delight of a child, but with a gaze that held a peculiar, unwavering focus. She strode directly towards it, her bare feet making soft, almost imperceptible sounds on the asphalt path. Other patients, mostly huddled near the food stalls or seated listlessly on folding chairs, barely registered her presence, much less her exposed state. The few staff members present were either distracted by the sparse crowd or hadn't yet processed the unfolding display.

She didn't climb onto one of the painted horses or swans. Instead, she used the carnival's position as a cover, a moment of chaos to exploit. The merry-go-round, spinning slowly with its repetitive, cheerful tune, offered a blind spot, a small pocket of activity that drew focus away from the more vulnerable sections of the facility perimeter.

With a sudden, astonishing burst of speed, she veered past the ride, not towards its entrance, but towards the less guarded, temporary fencing that enclosed the carnival area itself. It was a low chain-link barrier, hastily erected, meant more to delineate the space than to truly contain. Her slender frame, unhindered by clothing, moved with an agile economy. She was over it in a single fluid motion, a pale streak against the institutional green of the grounds.

An attendant, turning from a conversation with a fellow staff member, caught a glimpse of her. A flash of white against the distant foliage. A confused shout began to form but died in the throat. By the time the alarm was raised, she was already across the patch of manicured lawn, hurtling towards the more formidable, barbed-wire-topped fence that marked the true boundary of the facility.

But the carnival had necessitated a service gate, usually locked, often monitored, to be opened for deliveries and equipment. Today, in the relaxed atmosphere of the brief festivity, it had been left slightly ajar, or perhaps poorly secured. She must have known. She must have meticulously observed.

She was through it before anyone could react, a blur disappearing into the sparse woods that bordered the property. The distant, repetitive music of the merry-go-round, still playing its cheerful tune, became a strange, incongruous soundtrack to her sudden, silent freedom.

The two women, their faces a familiar mix of practiced patience and weary resignation, moved with the quiet efficiency of seasoned shepherds guiding a particularly stubborn lamb. No raised voices, no desperate pleas; just steady hands on her elbows, their steps echoing softly on the polished linoleum. She walked between them, her gait unhurried, a faint, almost imperceptible smile playing on her lips. After all, she'd done this before. Many times.

"We knew you'd be here," one of them murmured, less a reprimand and more a statement of simple fact.

This time, she hadn't attempted to orchestrate a diversion involving a precisely timed spill of dried beans in the communal dining hall, or, as in the now-legendary "Great Corn Capella" incident, a meticulously staged 'escape' involving a strategically placed bag of frozen vegetables in the industrial kitchen fryer. No, today's adventure had been far less dramatic, though no less baffling.

They'd found her in the staff breakroom, meticulously rearranging the sugar packets in the condiment caddy by color. She wasn't trying to escape the building, nor was she attempting to pilfer anything more valuable than a particularly plump shortbread biscuit from the staff-only stash. When asked, with a sigh, what exactly her objective had been, she merely looked up, her eyes twinkling with private amusement, and declared, "Order, my dear. Order."

It was a baffling moment, humorous, and entirely ridiculous, yet emblematic that on any given day, someone, somewhere was tipping the scales. Her departures weren't about freedom in the traditional sense; they were about a momentary, unassailable assertion of self, a tiny, defiant crack in the meticulously constructed order of things. She'd slip out during shift changes, during a particularly enthralling documentary in the day room, or simply whenever the mundane chaos of daily operations offered the slightest sliver of opportunity. The staff had learned not to chase, merely to anticipate her inevitable, brief, and utterly whimsical forays into the unauthorized.

No corn this time. Just two women escorting her back to her unit. They knew they would see her again, but never *when* they would see her. That rhythm belonged to her alone, a stubborn, beautiful, and utterly unpredictable beat in the heart of the facility. And frankly, a small, rebellious part of the staff, the part that occasionally dreamed of sneaking an extra ten minutes on their break, rather admired her for it.

# That Deaf Patient

The stale, institutional scent of Manteno Mental Health Center clung to everything, a mix of disinfectant, old linoleum, and something vaguely metallic. I was new, fresh out of whatever training was supposed to prepare me for this, and every corridor felt like a labyrinth designed to test my resolve. The patients were a spectrum of stories, whispered, shouted, or simply observed in the vacant stares that punctuated the long days. But there was one whose story I had to learn, letter by laborious letter.

His name was Gerald.

I first encountered him in at intake, a man perhaps in his thirties, with eyes that missed nothing, even as his ears registered almost nothing. He moved with a peculiar, deliberate grace, his hands often in motion, forming shapes only he seemed to understand. He'd been profoundly hearing impaired since childhood, a condition that had, over the decades, eroded not just his ability to hear, but his voice too. What must have once been words now emerged as breathy, high-pitched squeaks, sudden bursts of sound that carried no meaning, only the ghost of an effort. Sign language was his world, his lexicon, his lifeline.

My world, at that point, was still rooted in spoken words. I knew nothing of the silent dance of hands.

Our first real interaction was an exercise in mutual exasperation. I needed to ask him about his medication, a simple enough query for most, typically a five-minute exchange. For us, it became an epic. I started, as one does, by speaking. Gerald watched my lips, a flicker of something unreadable in his gaze before he shook his head slowly, a gesture of futility. That's when the gestures began.

My hands flailed, a clumsy, improvisational ballet of pointing to my mouth, then to his, then making a questioning shrug. Gerald, with a patience I mistook for understanding, offered back a cascade of fluid, intricate signs. My brain scrambled. It was like trying to decipher a complex poem written in a language I'd never heard, much less read.

Frustration rippled through me. Then, he offered the sign language alphabet. So, we began to spell. Each word became a monumental task. My fingers, stiff and awkward, fumbled through the shapes: A, B, C. His eyes tracked my every movement, sharp and appraising.

"M-E-D-I-C-A-T-I-O-N?" I spelled, fingers aching, my brow furrowed in concentration.

Gerald watched, then his own hands moved, swift and precise, correcting my clumsy 'T' into a perfect form, then spelling out an exasperated "Y-E-S." The process dragged on, thirty minutes melting away as we constructed rudimentary sentences, each one a small triumph wrested from the jaws of miscommunication.

It was frustrating, yes, but more than that, it was intimidating. He had a skill, a complete, sophisticated language, that I utterly lacked. He knew it. I could see the glint in his eye, the slight, almost imperceptible tilt of his head. He relished my ignorance, my slow, stumbling efforts. And then he laughed. It wasn't a cruel laugh, not entirely. It was a soundless, internal chortle that manifested as his shoulders shaking, his mouth opening in an unvoiced peal of amusement. He laughed at my clumsy 'G', at my stretched-out 'S', at the sheer, undeniable struggle painted across my face.

In that moment, standing in the sterile quiet of Manteno, Gerald, the deaf patient, held all the cards. He was the master, and I, the supposedly educated caregiver, was the bewildered student. It was infuriating, humbling, and, in a strange way, the beginning of something.

The laugh. It wasn't a cruel cackle, but a soft, almost wistful exhalation of amusement that seemed to bubble up from a deep, forgotten well. It grated on me, though. I was pouring every ounce of my effort into this, contorting my fingers into clumsy approximations of signs I'd only recently learned from an old manual, trying desperately to bridge the chasm between us. And he just... laughed. Was it at my ineptitude? Or was it something else entirely?

"Chicago," I signed again, slowly, exaggerating each movement. "Where in Chicago, Gerald?" I pointed to myself, then to him, then made a vague gesture of a house. He just smiled, a knowing glint in his eyes that made me feel even more like an amateur. He signed "C-H-I-C-A-G-O" again, with a flourish, then pointed to the ceiling, then swept his hand across the floor, then tapped his chest. My brain spun. High rise? Ground floor? His apartment? It was like trying to decipher an ancient riddle with half the pieces missing. The frustration was a hot coal in my gut, but beneath it, a stubborn flicker of something else – a fierce determination. I had to understand.

But the real question, the one that kept me up at night, circled back relentlessly: how was he admitted to Manteno? This wasn't just a matter of language; it was a matter of proper assessment, due process. In an era where even basic psychiatric understanding was evolving, and certainly before widespread awareness or accommodation for the deaf, how could a man who communicated solely through a language almost nobody here understood, be deemed "mentally ill" and committed? Who spoke his language well enough to interpret his thoughts, his fears, his needs? Who made the definitive diagnosis that landed him in this desolate place? The logic simply didn't hold.

My visits with Gerald continued, a Sisyphean task of fumbled signs and his enigmatic laughter. I kept trying, driven by that nagging question. Eventually, I knew I couldn't get the answer from Gerald directly, at least not yet. I needed to go to the source – or what passed for it here. I walked the long, echoing corridors to the administrative offices, the air thick with the smell of old paper and disinfectant. I requested Gerald's file.

The clerk, a woman named Agnes whose face seemed permanently set in an expression of weary resignation, eyed me over her spectacles. "Gerald?" she mused, flipping through a large, bound ledger. "Been here a long time, that one. File's probably in archives. Good luck."

"Archives" turned out to be a cavernous basement room, dimly lit and smelling of mildew and forgotten histories. Stacks of yellowed folders, tied with brittle string, lined shelves that stretched to the ceiling. It took two hours of dusty searching, my lungs burning, before I finally found it: a thick, dog-eared folder marked with Gerald's name and a faded admission date nearly two decades prior.

I carried it back to my office. The file was heavy, brittle, and felt like a repository of silent screams. The first few pages were standard: name, birth date, an address in Chicago – yes! – but no street number, just a district. And then, the admission notes. They read like a horror story of misinterpretation. "Patient exhibits severe mutism and disinterest in communication." "Displays repetitive hand gestures, possibly indicative of catatonia or delusional thought patterns." "Responds to spoken commands with blank stare, suggesting profound auditory hallucinations or complete withdrawal."

There was no mention of sign language. None. There were physician's notes signed by an anonymous psychiatrist. "Patient deemed unfit for independent living due to severe mental incapacitation. Requires permanent institutional care."

My eyes scanned the pages again, desperate for any indication of how this assessment was performed. How could they have possibly concluded any of this without understanding him? The final piece of documentation was a brief, almost dismissive note: "Admitted by concerned neighbor, following reports of patient's erratic behavior and inability to communicate."

A neighbor. Not family. A neighbor who apparently spoke no sign language, who only saw "erratic behavior" and "inability to communicate," and who then, somehow, had Gerald committed to Manteno. It was a monstrous injustice. I looked at the file, then back out my window towards the ward where Gerald would be.

His laugh, which I'd so misunderstood, resonated in my mind now not as mockery, but as a testament to an unbearable, decades-long irony. He wasn't laughing at me. He was laughing at the world, at the cruel, unseeing absurdity that had stolen his life. And I knew, with a sudden, overwhelming clarity, that I had to do more than just try to understand. I had to help him tell his story.

Gerald, a man whose presence was as quiet as the institution's demise. His patient file, like his demeanor, was unremarkable – a term often meant to indicate "normalcy" by omission, a way of saying he wasn't violent, wasn't prone to outburst, wasn't, in the most disruptive sense, "crazy." But unremarkable didn't mean normal. It meant isolated. Utterly, profoundly isolated. He could not have conversations with any other patients, nor staff. He was a silent island in a sea of babbling confusion, and the communication barrier was a wall none of us had found a way to breach.

He spent most of his waking hours in my office, a quiet fixture. He rarely spoke, and when he did, it was an unintelligible murmur. Yet, there was one gesture, a constant, repeated motion that became his signature: a hand shaped into a "C," often flashed quickly, definitively. It meant more than just Chicago. It was his anchor, his identity, a silent plea or declaration that spoke of home, of a past, of somewhere else.

I'd nod, offer a sympathetic smile, and acknowledge his "C," and for a moment, a thread of connection, however thin, would form between us.

Then came the day he sought to communicate something more complex, something beyond the simple identifier of the "C." He was agitated, a subtle tremor in his hands, his eyes fixed on me with an intensity I hadn't seen before. He signed something I didn't understand at all. Not even a guess. This simple gesture meant something I could not fathom. He placed his thumb and forefinger together, extended his arm, then, with his other hand pointed at a stack of papers that rested on my desk. I shrugged, my heart sinking. I felt helpless, a feeling that had become all too common in those final months. He wiggled his thumb and forefinger, still pressed together, his gaze unwavering, desperate. I slid my chair back and gestured toward the papers, giving him space, hoping he would play out whatever he was trying to communicate.

There are times when even smart, educated people overlook the obvious, when the very simplicity of a solution is obscured by the complexity of the problem. This was one of those times. I watched him – a man presumed entirely non-verbal, cut off from all meaningful exchange – pick up a pen. His grip was firm, deliberate. On a blank piece of paper, he wrote the words: "Chicago hospital."

The world tilted. My breath hitched. He could write! And he had known it all along! The revelation hit me like a physical blow, a wave of shock, then shame, then an overwhelming surge of elation. All this time, the years of silence, the isolation, and he possessed the key to his own inner world. The "C" suddenly unfurled its full meaning, no longer a mere city, but a gateway, a destination.

"Chicago hospital," I repeated, my voice hoarse. Gerald nodded vigorously, his eyes shining with a mixture of relief and triumph. It was a communication breakthrough that felt monumental, a tiny miracle amidst the dying embers of Manteno.

Over the next few weeks, the pen and paper became our bridge. Gerald, it turned out, wasn't just able to write; he was eloquent, precise, and utterly starved for connection. "Chicago hospital" wasn't just a place he remembered; it was where he'd been before Manteno, where he believed he belonged, where he had a record. He wrote about a doctor there who "understood," about a specific ward, about a time before the silence consumed him. He wasn't asking to return to a psychiatric facility, not exactly. He was asking for his history, for the threads of his identity that had been lost and tangled in the institutional shuffle. The "Chicago hospital" was his map back to himself.

We spent hours, Gerald patiently writing, me scribbling questions, his frustration melting away with each answered query. He told me, through careful script, about his hearing impairment, which had often been dismissed or misunderstood as a symptom of his mental health rather than a primary challenge. He detailed incidents where he'd been misjudged, mislabeled, simply because he couldn't hear, couldn't respond, couldn't clarify.

His "unremarkable" behavior, it turned out, was a fortress built of necessity, of resignation. He had learned the futility of trying to communicate when all his attempts were met with blank stares or misinterpretations. His silence wasn't a symptom; it was a strategy for survival in a world that hadn't given him the tools, or the chance, to be heard.

With Manteno's closure looming, this discovery was paramount. "Chicago hospital" was more than just a place; it was a lead, a direction for his future placement, a potential link to continuity of care, perhaps even to family who might still be looking. I used his written accounts, his clear, concise narratives, to advocate for him, to ensure his next placement understood his unique needs, to ensure his voice, finally, would not be silenced again.

Communication, with Gerald, was a battlefield of patience and guesswork. He'd meticulously arrange his few possessions, eat his meals with an almost ritualistic precision, and then, invariably, he would come to me, or to any staff member who seemed to have a moment, and point. He'd point an insistent finger towards the north, his brow furrowed with earnestness, and mouth the word, "Chicago."

At first, like everyone else, I assumed he meant the sprawling metropolis, the city of broad shoulders, perhaps a longing for family or a past life there. It was a common enough desire among our patients, a yearning for 'outside.' We'd nod, offer platitudes, explain that transfers were complicated, especially now, with the center closing. Gerald, however, was persistent. His "Chicago" wasn't a vague longing; it was a specific, urgent demand. His frustration, though silent, was palpable. He'd resort to drawing, crude stick figures and arrows, always pointing, always articulating that one word with a desperate hope in his eyes.

It took weeks, maybe longer, a slow, painstaking accretion of half-understood gestures, scribbled notes, and the occasional input from an older aide who remembered fragments of his file, to piece together the truth. Gerald didn't want to go to Chicago the city. His "Chicago" was Chicago Read Mental Health Center, a state hospital on the city's northwest side. More critically, Chicago Read had a dedicated unit for deaf and hearing-impaired patients, a place where Gerald had been understood, where he had access to ASL interpreters, to an environment tailored to his needs.

The revelation hit me with a dull ache of understanding and profound frustration. It wasn't the romantic yearning of a man for his hometown; it was the desperate plea of a displaced person for his actual home, his community. He wasn't pining for Lake Michigan; he was pining for the ability to communicate, to be seen, to belong.

How or why Gerald, a man who found his voice and his understanding in the specialized halls of Chicago Read, had been shunted to a sprawling, general facility like Manteno – especially one on its last legs, with no specialized deaf services – was a question that hung unanswered, a testament to the bewildering, sometimes cruel, logic of state bureaucracy. It seemed an act of profound dehumanization, to take a man from the one place where his disability was accommodated, and place him where it became an insurmountable barrier.

I tried, we all tried, to advocate for him, to explain his unique situation amidst the chaos of Manteno's closure. The paperwork was a nightmare, the system sluggish and overwhelmed. Every day, Gerald would find me, his "Chicago" a silent mantra on his lips, his hand pointing north. Each time, I felt a fresh stab of guilt and helplessness. He wasn't asking for the impossible; he was asking for what was rightfully his: an environment where he could thrive, or at least, exist with dignity and understanding.

In the scramble of those final weeks, as patients were dispersed to other centers, to group homes, or, in some cases, back to families, the last I saw of Gerald was a quick, harried transfer to a general unit in another facility. Did he ever make it back to his Chicago, his true Chicago? I never knew. But his silent, insistent plea, and the heartbreaking misunderstanding that underpinned it, remains one of the most poignant memories of my time in Manteno, a stark reminder of the individual lives caught in the impersonal grind of the system, desperately seeking a way back to where they belonged.

His "C" had found its meaning, not just as a city, but as a testament to the enduring human need to connect, to be understood, and the incredible, often overlooked, power of a simple pen and paper to bridge even the widest chasm of silence. He taught me that even in the most desolate places, the capacity for communication, for self-expression, can lie dormant, waiting for the simplest of opportunities to ignite.

# Lorraine

The ultrasound technician's voice was a warm, syrupy hum, a sound designed for joy. "Look at that little flutter, Lorraine! A strong heartbeat."

Every other expectant mother Lorraine had ever seen in magazines or on TV would have been beaming, perhaps tearing up. Lorraine felt a cold dread settle in her stomach, right where the tiny flutter was. This wasn't the celebrated 'achievement' society lauded. This was a biological fact, undeniable, terrifying.

For years, Lorraine had navigated the world with the steady anchor of medication. Thorazine, her quiet companion, had kept the whispers at bay, the shadows from coalescing into menacing figures. It had allowed her to work, to maintain a small, neat apartment, to pretend at a semblance of normalcy. But the moment the OB-GYN – a kind-faced woman with a concerned frown – delivered the verdict, the anchor was cut.

"The risks to the fetus... they're too significant, Lorraine," her doctor had explained gently, her voice full of a clinical compassion. "We have to take you off everything. It's for the baby's safety."

And just like that, Lorraine was adrift.

Soon thereafter she was admitted to Manteno.

The first week was a strange quiet, almost a honeymoon period. Then the buzzing started, faint at first, like a distant swarm of bees. It grew louder, a cacophony in her skull, drowning out the well-meaning advice of the few people who still spoke to her. "Are you eating enough, dear?" "You need to rest." "Just think of that precious little life inside you."

Lorraine would nod, feigning understanding, while her eyes darted to the shadows in the corner, convinced they were shifting, watching. The walls of the hospital, once a comforting cream, began to breathe, expanding and contracting with each beat of her turbulent heart. Her own reflection in the mirror was a stranger – gaunt, eyes wide with a fear that wasn't just about the baby, but about the world closing in.

The adoption agencies, like well-oiled machines, detected the scent of vulnerability. They called, they visited, their brochures glossy with smiling, hopeful couples. "We understand this is a difficult time, Lorraine," a Social Worker explained, her voice soothing but her gaze sharp, assessing. "Think of the beautiful life you could give this child. A stable home. Parents who have longed for a baby for years. It's an act of incredible selflessness."

The Social Worker had identified a couple, already vetted and approved for adoption. They couldn't conceive, for reasons undisclosed. For them, Lorraine wasn't a woman battling an invisible war; she was a vessel, an opportunity, a solution to their private sorrow. Her pregnancy, borne of circumstances the Social Worker dared not ask about, was their miracle.

They called it "saving" the child. And in the same breath, "saving" Lorraine from the grind of parenting, from the inevitable stigma of being a single mother, a mentally ill mother, a mother on the precipice of poverty. Her doctor, too, in her quiet way, had made her judgment. The fetus's well-being, its future, trumped Lorraine's present disintegration. The unseen chemical dance in Lorraine's brain was a secondary concern to the developing neural pathways of the child she carried.

Lorraine tried to explain. "The voices," she'd whispered to Brenda, clutching her belly. "They tell me... they tell me he's not real. Or that they want to take him."

The Social Worker had smiled, a little too brightly. "It's stress, dear. Pregnancy hormones can do wonders to a woman's mind. Just focus on the positive. Focus on the wonderful home you could provide for your baby."

The disconnect was a canyon. Society celebrated the ideal of pregnancy, the glowing mother, the achievement. But Lorraine was a living, breathing contradiction to that narrative. She was the inconvenient truth, the biological reality unpolished by magazines. Her pregnancy wasn't a baby shower, but a gauntlet of judgments.

As her belly swelled, so did the chaos in her mind. She started seeing patterns in the wallpaper, convinced they were coded messages. The refrigerator hummed with a malevolent intelligence. She rarely left her apartment, fearing the eyes that watched her from every window, every passing car.

Yet, amidst the terror, there was a nascent flicker. When the baby kicked, a strong, undeniable thump beneath her hand, something shifted. For a fleeting moment, the voices retreated, and a different reality asserted itself. This was real. This was a life. Her life, connected to this life.

One afternoon, sitting alone in the dim light of her living room, the adoption papers lay open on the coffee table. The adoptive parents' names, their perfect house, their hope, stared up at her. On the facing page, the legal clauses – the relinquishment, the parental rights.

A shadow detached itself from the corner, elongating, twisting. It whispered, "You can't. You'll ruin it. Like you ruin everything."

Lorraine closed her eyes, pressing her hands against her swollen abdomen. The baby kicked, a soft, insistent reminder. She remembered the flutter on the screen, the tiny heartbeat. It wasn't an achievement.

It wasn't a moral failing. It was just life. Raw. Unfiltered. And utterly, terrifyingly, hers.

The decision hung in the air, heavy and full of unasked questions. What would truly save this child? What would truly save Lorraine? And in a world that saw only black and white, who was left to navigate the agonizing grey?

The sterile, linoleum floor of the psychiatric unit seemed to amplify the echo of Lorraine's voice, a constant, simmering rage that had become the soundtrack to everyone's days. It wasn't a sudden eruption, but a slow, insidious build, a confluence of fragmented truths and dissonant voices that had been churning within her mind for months. Now, in her third trimester, the pressure had become unbearable, and the dam had broken.

Her anger was a palpable force, radiating from her like heat from a furnace. It was always there, a low hum that could quickly escalate into a roaring inferno. Every interaction was a potential battleground. A nurse's gentle inquiry about her appetite would be met with a sneer and a barbed accusation of being in league with the doctors who had "done this to her." A fellow patient offering a sympathetic nod would be met with suspicion and a shouted denouncement of their supposed ulterior motives.

Lorraine's words were sharp, precise weapons, designed to wound and isolate. She accused, she blamed, she dissected every perceived slight, every imagined betrayal, each with a chilling conviction that made it difficult for anyone to refute. Her accusations weren't wild ramblings; they were often laced with disturbing fragments of reality, distorted and twisted into a narrative of persecution. This made her more terrifying than the overtly delusional patients. While their flights of fancy were sometimes easy to dismiss, Lorraine's rage felt rooted in a twisted logic that was harder to untangle.

The staff, accustomed to the various manifestations of mental illness, found themselves walking on eggshells. They avoided her area of the common room, their conversations hushed when she was within earshot. Even the most seasoned nurses, who had seen and heard it all, began to wear a weary, defeated look. A few, driven by concern for both Lorraine and the fragile peace of the unit, had cautiously approached the attending psychiatrist.

Her psychiatrist, a man whose calm demeanor was usually a steady anchor in the storm of the unit, looked troubled. He knew the history. Before the pregnancy, Lorraine had been on a regimen of antipsychotics that had effectively muted the cacophony in her mind, rendering her lucid, compliant, and, most importantly, quiet. But the current protocol, aiming for the least amount of interference during pregnancy, had seen those medications gradually reduced and eventually discontinued. The intention had been to let her find her own equilibrium, but her mind, it seemed, had chosen a different path.

Lorraine herself was a stark contrast to the quiet, subdued woman she had been months ago. Her face, usually pale and drawn, was now flushed with a perpetual flush of fury. Her eyes, once holding a flicker of vulnerability, now blazed with an unyielding resentment. She was not physically aggressive. She didn't throw punches or shatter furniture. Her aggression was verbal, a torrent of venom that could strip a person bare. It was the venom, the unwavering intensity of her anger, that made her so intimidating. She stood tall, her pregnant belly a testament to the life growing within her, a life she seemed to resent with every fiber of her being.

The air around her crackled with unspoken threats. Even when she wasn't speaking, her silence was heavy with anticipation, as if she were gathering strength for her next verbal assault. The other patients, once willing to connect, now treated her like a volatile force of nature, something to be observed from a safe distance, their own peace dependent on not drawing her attention. Lorraine, trapped within the confines of her own mind, a maelstrom of conflicting thoughts and overwhelming emotions, was becoming a solitary island of rage, her voice the only thing that seemed to anchor her to the world, albeit a world she was determined to burn down with her words.

Lorraine, her face a mask of exhaustion and anticipation, lay on the gurney, the rhythmic thrum of her contractions echoing not just in her body, but in the very air around her. It was a sound that, for the usually bustling staff, heralded not just another birth, but a moment of profound relief. Peace on the ward, they whispered, a hushed excitement rippling through the corridors.

The adoptive parents, a young couple whose faces radiated a tender hope, had been on standby for weeks. Today, they were summoned not just to witness the arrival of "their" child, but to become its immediate guardians. The umbilical cord, that natural, life-sustaining link, felt more like a countdown timer, a fragile thread whose severance held the promise of a swift departure, an immediate transition. The anxiety clinging to them was palpable, a silent prayer for a smooth, swift delivery.

Lorrane was wheeled into a private room, a staged tableau of impending birth. She lay on the gurney, her moans growing louder, the pain a physical force bearing down on her. The room held the doctor, a man whose gentle demeanor belied the gravity of the situation, the expectant adoptive parents, Lorraine, and me, an observer in this intimate, yet strangely public, drama. The doctor, a paragon of his oath, offered no immediate relief for Lorraine's escalating pain.

But as Lorriane's body faltered, her will seemingly waning, the situation escalated. The contractions, powerful and relentless, were met with a stillness that defied biological imperative. Lorraine did not push.

Instead, a desperate, strangled cry escaped her lips, a sound raw with pain and a resistance no one understood. The doctor, his brow furrowed, his usual calm fraying at the edges, found himself at a moral and ethical precipice. The life of the baby, already on the cusp of existence, hung in the balance. The consequences of inaction loomed, horrific and undeniable.

Then, a flicker of movement. Lorraine's legs crossed, a tight, involuntary clench. Why? Was it a desperate attempt to staunch the searing pain? A primal act of self-preservation? Or a silent, desperate rebellion against the unfolding certainty? The reason remained a mystery, a fleeting enigma in the whirlwind of birth.

But the doctor, his face etched with a harsh pragmatism, no longer had the luxury of contemplation. He produced a scalpel, its gleam catching the sterile light. His voice, though quiet, cut through the rising tide of sound and fear. "You push," he stated, his gaze unwavering, "or I cut you open." The choice, stark and brutal, was laid bare. The peace the ward had anticipated felt impossibly distant, replaced by a chilling ultimatum.

The sterile scent of antiseptic was usually a comfort to Lorraine. It meant order, cleanliness, the quiet hum of machines keeping tiny lives stable. But today, it felt cloying, suffocating. Her own body, a landscape of exhaustion and ache, was the counterpoint to the pristine room. She'd pushed. The word felt too small, too light for the monumental effort that had just concluded.

And then, there it was. A squalling, wrinkled miracle. A baby. Hands, so small they could fit in the palm of Lorraine's own, flailed with surprising strength. A shock of dark hair, damp and clinging to a tiny head. The nurse, efficient and gentle, cleaned the infant, her movements practiced and swift. Then came the swaddling – a firm, secure cocoon that seemed to instantly calm the little protests.

The door opened, not with the usual hushed urgency of a medical emergency, but with a soft click. Two figures stood there, their faces a mixture of apprehension and overwhelming hope. They were the adoptive parents. Lorraine had met them briefly before, seen the quiet strength in their eyes, the tremor in their hands when they'd spoken about the baby they so desperately wanted.

The nurse, with a knowing smile, approached them. The baby, now a perfectly formed bundle, was carefully placed into the waiting arms. A gasp, soft and almost reverent, escaped the woman. The man's arm went immediately around her, his gaze fixed on the tiny being nestled against her chest. Tears, no longer held back, traced paths down their cheeks.

They thanked the doctor, their voices thick with emotion. The doctor, a woman of quiet competence, offered a few words of advice, a gentle reassurance. Then, their eyes found Lorraine.

Lorraine was an observer. A witness. Her job was not to hold, to nurture, to embark on the lifelong journey of parenting. Her job was to facilitate. To make the space, to guide, to ensure the safe passage of a life from one set of hands to another. She had done her part. She had cleaned the room, prepared the equipment, monitored the vital signs, and in the quiet moments between the doctor's instructions and the nurse's ministrations, she had simply been there. A steady presence in a moment of profound transition.

The adoptive mother's gaze met hers, and in those eyes, Lorraine saw a world of gratitude, unburdened by the physical reality of childbirth, but acutely aware of the vulnerability of the moment. "Thank you," the woman whispered, her voice catching. "Thank you for... everything."

The man nodded, his own eyes shining. "We're so grateful. Truly."

Lorraine offered a soft smile, a gesture that felt inadequate for the enormity of what had just occurred. She felt a pang, not of regret, but of a quiet, peculiar sadness. A life had begun, a family had been formed, and she, who had been so intimately involved in the mechanics of it all, was already receding. A chapter closed, a story continued elsewhere.

They left, the three of them – the new parents and their precious cargo, a beacon of hope stepping out into the world. The door clicked shut behind them, leaving Lorraine in the quiet aftermath. The sterile scent still hung in the air, but now, it carried a faint echo of whispered thanks, of overwhelming joy, and of the silent, profound privilege of bearing witness.

Her world had been a kaleidoscope of jagged edges and distorted echoes for weeks. A fragile vessel adrift in a storm, Lorraine had resisted everything – food, comfort, and most vehemently, the pills that promised to tame the roaring chaos inside her head. There had been a frantic push-and-pull with the medical staff, a period of foggy, terrified compliance, followed by a fierce, desperate refusal, until the exhaustion of it all left her too weak to fight.

Soon thereafter, her medication regime was re-started. The nurse, with eyes that held both unwavering calm and a deep understanding, would bring the small plastic cup each morning and evening. The first few times, Lorraine had clutched her jaw, the thought of swallowing anything feeling like an insurmountable task. But the nurse was patient. She didn't push, merely waited, a glass of water shimmering beside the small, potent tablets. Slowly, tentatively, Lorraine would take them. The chalky taste was an anchor, pulling her back to the present, however unwelcome.

Gradually, she settled into the hospital routine. The relentless static in her mind began to quiet, replaced by the mundane rhythms of the ward. The distant clang of the food trolley, the hushed consultations outside her door, the soft footsteps of the night nurse checking on sleeping patients – these sounds, once merely part of the overwhelming din, now took on a distinct, almost comforting pattern.

Her eyes, formerly darting and unfocused, began to linger. On the faded floral pattern of the curtains, on the way the afternoon sun sliced across the linoleum floor, illuminating motes of dust dancing in the air. She started to recognize faces: the kind, weary lines around the nurse's eyes, the perpetually bewildered expression of Mr. Harrison down the hall, the crisp, professional demeanor of her psychiatrist during ward rounds.

She learned the unspoken language of the hospital: the specific chime of the medication cart, the scent of antiseptic that clung to the air, the predictable ebb and flow of visitors. Mornings meant the brisk energy of shift change, afternoons brought the quiet lull of rest periods, and evenings descended with a gentle, drowsy hum. She began to anticipate.

The food, initially unappetizing, became sustenance. She felt the warmth of her blanket, the coolness of her pillow, little sensations that had been lost beneath the weight of her despair. There were still bad days, moments when the shadows threatened to creep back in, but they were fewer, shorter, and less potent. The medication wasn't a magic wand, but a steadying hand, a subtle re-calibration of the inner compass that had spun wildly off course.

Lorraine remained in the quiet, long after the door had closed. The rhythms of the ward resumed—the distant clang of the food trolley, the soft murmur of nurses—but something had shifted. She was no longer the storm, nor the vessel, nor the cautionary tale. She was the witness. The one who endured, who refused, who recalibrated. And though the child she bore now belonged to another story, unfolding somewhere beyond these walls, Lorraine's own remained—etched in the linoleum light, in the dust motes she had learned to watch, in the chalky taste of survival. Not erased. Not redeemed. Just present. Still here.

And when the adoptive parents offered visitation, Lorraine declined. The cord had already been cut—not just from her child, but from the rhythm of her body, the pulse of her refusal, the storm she had survived.

# Marcus

The late afternoon sun, a muted smear of orange through the perpetually grimy windows of Manteno State Hospital, cast long, distorted shadows across the linoleum floor. It was a light that never truly reached the corners, perpetually battling the institutional pallor of pale green walls and scuffed metal furniture. This was the domain of the "managed," the "bridged," the ones deemed too dangerous for society's everyday rhythm, yet not quite lost to the absolute void that was Chester.

The patients at Manteno weren't criminals in the conventional sense. Not yet, anyway. They were the Unfit to Stand Trial, the Not Guilty By Reason of Insanity, the ones whose minds had fractured in ways that made the legal system pause, to declare them incapable of comprehending their actions or defending themselves. They were a constant, unsettling reminder of the thin, often invisible, line between sanity and its absence, a line they had demonstrably crossed.

The forensic wards were a peculiar purgatory. They weren't the stark, formidable fortresses of Chester Mental Health Center, where the truly lost, the irrevocably dangerous, were held under an unyielding gaze. Chester was the end of the line, the place where hope was a cruel joke. Manteno, on the other hand, was a transitional space, a holding pen where the courts could satisfy their need for containment without resorting to the ultimate isolation. It was a judgment call, a calculation of risk versus resource. These individuals, while possessing troubling histories, were deemed manageable. Medium-security manageable.

Marcus was one of the "high-risk" patients, his file probably thicker than most. There had been an incident, a violent outburst that had landed him here, but the doctors had deemed him stable enough for Manteno's gentle, yet firm, embrace. He would spend hours in the recreation room, meticulously stacking worn playing cards, his brow furrowed in concentration. Then, without warning, he'd erupt into a peal of laughter, a sound so incongruous it sent shivers down the spines of the staff and the other patients alike.

The staff here were not gladiators, nor were they wardens. They were caretakers, trained to de-escalate, to observe, to administer medication, and to maintain a fragile equilibrium. They navigated the labyrinth of damaged minds with a blend of empathy and detachment, a skill honed through necessity. They understood that these patients were not simply "crazy," but individuals whose internal landscapes had been irrevocably scarred by trauma, illness, or circumstance.

The grounds of Manteno State Hospital, though vast and dotted with the melancholy beauty of older trees, could feel suffocatingly small at times. For Marcus, however, they were a stage. He navigated the familiar paths with a practiced ease, a phantom limb of his former life, perhaps, or a deep-seated understanding of the human psyche. He was a fixture, as reliable as the afternoon sun filtering through the leaves, a man often seen walking the grounds, sitting on a particular bench that offered a good vantage point, or engaged in earnest conversation.

His companions varied. Sometimes it was another patient, their eyes vacant or alight with a shared delusion, their responses a fragmented echo of Marcus's own carefully crafted narrative. More often, it was staff, their faces etched with the weariness of a thousand similar encounters, their conversations punctuated by the polite but firm boundaries they were trained to maintain.

The truth, the one that flickered just beneath the surface of his affable demeanor, was that Marcus was charmingly manipulative. It wasn't a crude, obvious tactic. It was far more subtle, a delicate probing of vulnerabilities, an artful calibration of appeal. He had an uncanny knack for ascertaining who around him possessed a pliable spirit, those who might be persuaded to grant his seemingly simple requests. Conversely, he seemed to know, instinctively, those who simply denied engagement, whose defenses were too robust or whose internal compass pointed them away from the siren song of his requests.

My path, in the impersonal rhythm of the institution, had crossed with Marcus on several occasions. It was inevitable, given the shared space. Our conversations, without fail, began with a request. It started small, as all good manipulations do. A cigarette, often. Sometimes a small sum of money, just enough for something he claimed to desperately need – a particular snack, a book from the commissary. Later, the requests would shift, becoming slightly more complex, still framed in a way that seemed utterly reasonable, a minor inconvenience for a fellow human.

He was a master of the gentle art of the ask. He'd lean in, his eyes earnest, his voice a low, persuasive murmur. He'd weave a brief, compelling narrative to justify his need, a tale that rarely felt entirely fabricated, but rather a carefully embellished truth. He'd highlight the shared humanity, the simple act of kindness, the minor obligation we all owed to one another, especially within these walls.

And I, like many others, was the recipient of this well-honed charm. He never succeeded, not a single time. My own internal compass, perhaps, was calibrated to recognize the scent of a carefully constructed appeal. Or perhaps it was simply the ingrained professional distance that prevented me from crossing that particular line.

But he always tried. That was the enduring constant. The persistence, the unwavering belief that this time, this time, the carefully chosen words and the earnest gaze would finally break through. He would finish his request, his eyes holding mine, waiting. And I would deliver my familiar, polite refusal.

Even in those rejections, there was a strange kind of interaction. He didn't typically react with anger or frustration. Instead, a subtle shift would occur. The earnestness might dim slightly, replaced by a flicker of something else – disappointment, yes, but also a subtle recalculation. He'd nod, perhaps a small, tight smile, and then, with a disarming grace, he'd pivot.

"I get it," he might say, his tone still light, "I understand. Thanks." And he'd move on, his gaze already scanning for his next mark, his next stage, his next carefully orchestrated attempt to bend the world, just a little, to his will, within the confines of Manteno's ever-watchful grounds.

The air in the unit always hummed with a low-grade tension, a static electricity of unspoken resentments and carefully managed desires. Most staff, were too busy navigating the treacherous currents of patient moods and administrative demands to give much thought to the subtle power plays unfolding around them. They just put their heads down, did the work, and tried to make it through the day. It was easier to believe, in those quieter moments, that they held some sway, some leverage, over the inscrutable Marcus and the others under his... influence. A small, comforting illusion, really.

But there was one, a particular staff member, whose need for Marcus' approval was a gaping maw that seemed to swallow all reason. His eyes, always darting towards Marcus, seeking that flicker of acknowledgment, that nod of approval, were a constant, unsettling presence. It was this man, driven by a desperation I still can't fathom, who brought the gun to the unit. And not just any gun, but a loaded one. The weight of it, I imagine, must have felt both terrifying and exhilarating in his trembling hands.

The details of what happened next are a smear of fragmented whispers and secondhand accounts. I wasn't there. I did not work on that unit.

But the story, as it's been pieced together, paints a chilling picture. Marcus, ever the collector of vulnerabilities, had asked to inspect the weapon. And this staff member, in his desperate bid to please, had complied. He'd handed it over. The cold, metallic weight of it, passed from one unsteady hand to another, instantly shifted the landscape of power. Suddenly, the illusion of control we staff had clung to evaporated. In Marcus' hands, the gun wasn't just a tool of intimidation; it was a stark, undeniable manifestation of leverage. A promise of consequences.

The next thing I knew, there were sirens. Not the distant wail of a passing ambulance, but a chorus of flashing lights and authoritative shouts. Seven cop cars. Seven. They formed a silent, formidable perimeter around the building, their red and blue lights painting strobe-like patterns on the brickwork.

From my vantage point, blocks away, even at that distance, I could sense the shift. The hum of the unit was gone, replaced by an abrupt, deafening silence. Marcus, at gunpoint – his gunpoint – had ordered everyone out. Staff, patients, the entire fragile ecosystem of the unit, spilling onto the pavement under the cold, indifferent gaze of the law. And he, Marcus, remained inside. Alone.

My supervisor, Ed, always creative in de-escalation and never one to let a patient trump his military training, deployed me to the forensic unit so "negotiate" with Marcus. I said, "Ed, that's what cops are for." Ed, with that infuriatingly calm, 'I know best' smile, had replied, "You know him. You can reason with him. Convince him to give you the gun, and walk out. The cops will do the rest."

Terrible plan, I thought, as the two of us walked toward the forensic unit. Absolutely insane. This would end poorly, I thought. My heart hammered a frantic rhythm against my ribs.

"You know him," Ed's words echoed. And he was right, in the most inconvenient way possible. I knew him only because Marcus had tried to manipulate me on several occasions, but never successfully. I had always managed to talk him down before. But a gun? That was a new, terrifying variable.

The forensic unit was a fortress within a fortress. Steel doors, reinforced glass, coded keypads. Security guards, usually a comforting presence, now stood by, grim-faced, riot shields at the ready, their body armor glinting under the harsh fluorescent lights.

Ed, oblivious, merely clapped me on the shoulder. "Just like talking him out of that 'alien invasion' fantasy, right? Except this time, the aliens brought a firearm." He even chuckled. I didn't. My mouth was dry enough to sand wood.

We reached Marcus's section. The corridor was empty, unnaturally quiet. The only sound was the low hum of the ventilation system and the distant, muffled chatter of a police radio. Marcus's door, usually ajar or frequently opened by staff, was now firmly shut, a single, dark eye staring from the peephole.

"Marcus?" I called out, my voice betraying a tremor I desperately tried to suppress. "It's me. I'm here to talk."

A pause. Then, a raw, guttural voice, thick with paranoia, responded. "I ain't going to Chester!"

Ed, standing a safe ten feet behind me, raised an eyebrow. "See? He knows you. Just engage him."

I shot Ed a glare that could curdle milk. "Marcus, please. Just open the door. Let's talk face to face."

A click. The door slowly, agonizingly, creaked open a sliver. I peered inside. The room was a disaster zone: overturned furniture, scattered papers. And Marcus, crouched in a corner, eyes wide and bloodshot, clutching something dark and metallic to his chest. It was a pistol, an old service revolver, probably smuggled in by a visitor or a profoundly incompetent staff member – a question for later. Right now, it was a very real, very present threat.

"Nobody's trying to trick you, Marcus," I said, my voice carefully modulated, trying to project calm I didn't feel. "We just want to make sure you're safe."

"Safe?" He barked a laugh, chilling and devoid of humor. "Safe from the truth? Never!" He pointed the gun, not directly at me, but at the wall beside my head. The movement was jerky, unpredictable. My heart leaped into my throat.

"Marcus, that's not safe. Let's put that down, okay?" I took a slow, deliberate step forward, extending my hands, palms open, in a gesture of peace. "Just hand it to me. No one's going to hurt you."

"He's escalating," Ed muttered from behind me, unnecessarily. "Try the 'I understand' approach."

I ignored Ed. "No, Marcus, I'm not. I'm just Brian. Remember? We talked about your mother's rose garden. We talked about your blueprints. You trusted me."

A flicker of something crossed his face, a momentary crack in the paranoia. Nostalgia? Recognition? Hope? It was fleeting.

Every muscle in my body tensed. This was it. The moment I became a statistic. I could almost hear the headlines: "Man Shot During De-escalation Attempt."

My mind raced. Ed's 'plan' was dissolving into chaos. The gun was inches from me. I could see the cold, dark bore of the barrel. Marcus's finger was still twitching. I had to do something, anything. I remembered a trick from a de-escalation seminar, something about breaking patterns, confusing the attacker.

"Marcus," I said, my voice surprisingly steady, "you're right."

His eyes, wide and manic, narrowed slightly. "What?"

"You're right," I repeated, louder, injecting a strange urgency into my tone. "They are coming. And they do want your thoughts. But this," I gestured wildly at the gun, "this is what they want you to have. They planted it! It's a tracking device! They want you to make noise, so they know exactly where you are!"

It was a desperate, insane gamble, twisting his own delusion against him. Ed behind me made a small choking sound, probably at the sheer audacity, or stupidity, of my words.

Marcus stared at the gun in his hand, then back at me. A deep furrow appeared in his brow, warring with the paranoia. "A tracking device?" he whispered, his voice losing some of its edge. "They... they put it in my hand?"

"Exactly!" I pressed, taking another careful step. "They want you to use it. They want you to betray yourself. But you're smarter than that, Marcus. You're brilliant. You know how to outsmart them."

He looked at the weapon as if seeing it for the first time, not as a shield, but as a trap. His grip, though still tight, faltered. "Outsmart... them?"

"Yes! Give it to me, Marcus. I'll dispose of it. I'll make sure they can't trace you through it. I'll protect your thoughts. You trust me, right?"

He looked at me, then at the gun, then back at me. The internal war raged visible across his face. The tremor in his hands increased, but this time, it felt like confusion more than rage.

Then, with an abruptness that made me flinch, he thrusted the gun forward. "Take it! Take it! Get it away from me before they hear!"

My fingers closed around the cold metal. It was heavier than I expected. For a split second, I feared he would pull me forward, or pull the trigger, or both. But he just stumbled back, collapsing onto his bed, his chest heaving, his eyes still wide with terror, but the immediate threat now gone.

I quickly disarmed the weapon, ejected the magazine, and slid the components to a waiting security guard who instantly secured them. Marcus, meanwhile, was already being gently approached by the crisis intervention team, his paranoia having shifted from external threat to the internal 'tracking device' he thought he'd just relinquished.

I stepped out of the unit, my legs shaking so badly I could barely stand. Ed rushed over, his face pale beneath his usual tan. "Holy hell, Brian, that was... brilliant. Utterly insane, but brilliant." He was trying to sound casual, but his voice cracked.

"You're lucky I'm not going to punch you," I rasped, leaning against the sterile wall, trying to catch my breath. The smell of antiseptic now clung to my clothes, a grim reminder of how close I'd come. My hands were still trembling.

"So, about that 'cops do the rest' part?" Ed asked, ever the pragmatist.

"Yeah. The cops can take it from here," I said, pushing off the wall. "After I get a very, very strong coffee. And maybe a new supervisor. Because Ed, your brilliance almost got me killed."

He just gave me that infuriating, knowing smile. "But it didn't, did it? You know him. You can reason with him."

I just walked away, leaving him to explain the 'tracking device' element of the successful de-escalation to the police. My plan, I thought, had been terrible. His, however, was worse. And yet, somehow, we'd survived it. I knew one thing for sure: next time Ed deployed me to 'negotiate,' I was bringing my own tactical gear. And a very large raise request.

“Ed? I taking tomorrow off. And the next day. And the next day. And the day after that...”

Ed laughed. “Good job.”

But, crazier than all of that, the staff person was fired. He appealed to the union. He was reinstated with back pay.

I don't know whether Marcus' behavior or the staff person's reinstatement were more disturbing.

Later that week, Marcus was transferred to Chester Mental Health Center. The decision came swiftly, almost bureaucratically, as if the breach had simply triggered a protocol. No ceremony. No farewell. Just a van, a form, and the quiet disappearance of a man who once held the unit in his trembling hands. Chester—the end of the line, where shimmer becomes silence.

Once a patient is transferred, they're rarely remembered. The system doesn't mourn—it resets. Marcus became a line item, a closed file, a name that no longer echoed in the staff lounge. And that, somehow, was more terrifying than the gun.

**Marvin**

The first time I saw Marvin, he was a ghost in the periphery of Manteno State Hospital. Fifteen years. The number echoed in my mind like a misplaced chime as I observed him. Fifteen years he'd been a fixture within these linoleum halls, a quiet testament to a life lived in shades of muted grey.

He wasn't the kind of patient who commanded attention, not by choice or by nature. There was no fiery glint in his eyes, no tremor of unease in his posture. Marvin was soft-spoken, his words few and carefully chosen, delivered in a tone that barely disturbed the air. His movements were deliberate, his steps silent on the worn floors, as if he were trying to leave the smallest possible footprint on the world.

I watched him interact with the nurses, with the other patients. He'd nod in acknowledgment, offer a brief, almost imperceptible smile, and then retreat back into himself. He never sought out conversation, and rarely initiated it. When asked a direct question, his answers were concise, devoid of elaboration. It beggared belief that this man, so gentle and unassuming, required the constant oversight of Manteno.

The records stated his admission date, a sterile fact that masked a story I suspected was far more personal and perhaps, less justifiable. His parents were gone, he'd mentioned once, a fleeting statement as if acknowledging a weather pattern. No siblings, no relatives ever visited. The absence of any familial connection or external support system felt like a gaping hole, a missing piece of the puzzle that explained his permanent residence.

But looking at Marvin, at the quiet way he'd sit by the window, watching the world go by without complaint, I couldn't shake the feeling that his placement was less about his incapacitation and more about the convenience of others. Someone, somewhere, had made a decision that deemed Manteno the most suitable, perhaps the easiest, solution for Marvin. A solution that removed him from view, from the complexities of life outside these walls, without any apparent necessity for the rigorous supervision he received.

He wasn't a danger. The staff knew it, the other patients knew it, and I, in my brief time observing him, certainly knew it. He was not a risk to himself, nor was he a threat to anyone else. He was simply present, a quiet observer in the grand, often bewildering, theater of Manteno. He existed within its confines, often overlooked, never requiring the urgent attention that other residents might necessitate. He was just Marvin, a man who talked and walked quietly, a man whose presence was a constant, gentle hum in the vast silence of the hospital, a silence that felt both chosen and imposed.

Marvin did not smoke. But, every week he announced he was walking to the canteen to purchase a carton of cigarettes. Every week he returned without a carton of cigarettes. I didn't think much of it. Maybe he changed his mind? Maybe the canteen didn't have his brand? He wasn't a smoker anyway.

The next week he repeated what would become a weekly ritual: announcement that he was going out to purchase a cartoon of cigarettes, return without the cigarettes. Something wasn't right.

I asked Marvin why he left to purchase cigarettes, but never returned with cigarettes. Not a pack, let alone a carton. And that's when Marvin told me, calmly "Somebody stole my cigarettes." He didn't protest. It was, to him, a fact.

And it made sense. In a place where luxury items were based in an economy of beg, borrow, or steal, Marvin was believable. We weren't in a prison, not officially, but the facility where we worked felt like one sometimes. Long shifts, minimal contact with the outside world, and a strictly controlled supply chain meant that even a candy bar could become a bargaining chip. Cigarettes, as a high-demand item, were practically currency.

But something still gnawed at me. How could his cigarettes be stolen every single time? Before he even got them back to unit, or—more perplexing—before he even left the canteen? Because he always returned with empty hands. Not even a crumpled wrapper, not a single filter. Zero evidence of a transaction, let alone a theft.

The next Tuesday, Marvin stood up from his console, stretched, and made his usual announcement, his voice completely devoid of any emotion that might betray the strangeness of his ritual. "Right, off to the canteen. Need to pick up a carton of cigarettes."

A few of the other technicians grunted in response. Old Man Henderson, who perpetually smelled of stale coffee and desperation, perked up. "What brand you getting, Marvin? My usual's been out."

Marvin didn't even look at him. "Just the usual. Whatever they have." He moved with the slow, deliberate pace of a man undertaking a monumental task, or perhaps, a man just going through the motions.

This time, I didn't let it go. "Mind if I walk with you, Marvin?" I asked, trying to sound casual as I pushed back from my own screen.

He paused, a flicker of something unreadable in his eyes, then gave a curt nod. "OK."

The walk to the canteen, or rather, what passed for one, was a short affair. We traversed impeccably manicured lawns, each blade of grass seemingly aligned with military precision. Yet, beneath the veneer of serenity, the air thrummed with the distant, insistent drone of servers. It was a constant, low-grade hum, a pervasive reminder of our gilded cage, our isolation from the world beyond these walls.

The "canteen" itself was a misnomer. It wasn't a place for communal meals or social gathering. It was simply the administrative building, housing a sterile, small alcove where one could procure essential, if rudimentary, items. Marvin, his movements practiced and deliberate, approached the woman behind the counter. He produced a crisp twenty-dollar bill from his worn wallet, its edges softened by countless transactions. "Carton of cigarettes," he stated, his voice a low rumble.

The woman, her face a mask of practiced indifference, seemed unsurprised. This routine, I gathered, was not uncommon. She retrieved a carton of cigarettes from beneath the counter, the cellophane crinkling softly as she handed it over. The transaction was swift, efficient, and devoid of any warmth.

As we began our return journey across the verdant expanse, Marvin abruptly stopped. He turned towards a man I'd never seen before. In this place, that was hardly remarkable; we housed a multitude of patients, each with their own story, their own history etched onto their faces. This man was just another transient figure in our controlled landscape. Then, with an almost casual gesture, I watched Marvin hand the carton of cigarettes to this stranger and resume his walk, his stride heavy.

"Marvin," I called out, my voice laced with a bewilderment that mirrored the confusion churning within me. "You just gave away your cigarettes."

Marvin paused, turning his head slightly, his gaze meeting mine for a fleeting moment. "He stole them," he replied, his tone flat, devoid of emotion.

The mystery, already intricate, tightened its grip. The simple act of purchasing cigarettes had unraveled into something far more complex. Was Marvin acting as a clandestine courier, a conduit between this anonymous man and the limited offerings of the "canteen"? Was he coerced, indebted, or simply playing some unseen game within the confines of our institutional existence? The hum of the servers seemed to amplify, as if to drown out the growing questions that now echoed in my mind.

The fluorescent lights of the hospital hummed a familiar, monotonous tune. I watched Marvin from my office window, a stoic figure moving with practiced ease through the common areas. He'd just emerged from the commissary, a small paper bag clutched in his hand. The man he was with, a hulking individual named Jim who radiated an aura of simmering resentment, was already lighting up a cigarette pulled directly from that very bag.

My gut twisted. This was the third week in a row. I excused myself, the click of my heels on the linoleum a stark counterpoint to the muffled drone of the prison. I intercepted Marvin before he disappeared into the labyrinthine corridors.

"Did that man threaten you?" My voice was deliberately low, a careful balance of concern and authority.

Marvin shook his head, his gaze unreadable as he sidestepped me, already moving away. I didn't let him go. I caught his arm, gently but firmly.

"Marvin," I repeated, my voice a little sharper this time. "Why are you buying cigarettes for this man?"

He paused, turning to face me, his expression unchanging. "He steals them."

The words hung in the air, a non-sequitur that left me reeling. Steals them? From whom? From the commissary? Was this some convoluted code for Jim extorting payment from him? Or a pre-arranged agreement, a silent understanding between two men I barely knew? Marvin's quiet compliance, his almost robotic acceptance of these weekly transactions, was more unsettling than any overt act of defiance.

"Marvin," I pressed, trying a different tack, a more direct accusation. "He didn't steal them. You gave them to him. You bought them."

He offered no response. Instead, he held the door open to his designated unit, a silent invitation for me to enter. I declined, watching as he then turned and disappeared into his room, a soft click indicating he was settling in for his afternoon nap.

Back in my office, the questions churned. Where was Marvin, a man with no income, no outside connections, acquiring the funds to purchase packs of cigarettes week after week? Who was the architect of this clandestine operation? And why this elaborate charade, this insistence that the cigarettes were 'stolen'? It was a puzzle with too many missing pieces, each one hinting at a deeper, more complex narrative unfolding within these walls.

The following week, as predictable as the sunrise filtering through the barred windows, Marvin stood up from his assigned seat. There was no announcement, no fanfare. But I knew. My instincts, honed by years in this environment, screamed where he was headed, and more importantly, who he was meeting. This time, I wouldn't let it play out.

I intercepted him again, before he could even approach the commissary entrance. "Marvin," I said, my tone firm, cutting through the usual prison chatter. "Skip the canteen. You're playing basketball today."

He registered my words with a characteristic shrug, a subtle shift in his posture. Then, to my surprise, he followed me, his feet carrying him towards the gymnasium.

The basketball court was a stark contrast to the grey monotony of the common areas. The air was thick with the scent of sweat and the squeak of sneakers. A pick-up game was underway, a flurry of activity. Marvin, however, stood at the periphery, an island of stillness in the energetic chaos. He displayed no discernible interest in the game, no flicker of engagement.

My objective, of course, was to break through his passive existence, to elicit some reaction, some sign of the man beneath the stoic facade. In an attempt to draw him in, to make him a part of something, I retrieved a stray basketball. I moved towards him, the ball in my hands.

I passed it to him, gently. A bounce pass. It was meant to be a simple, approachable gesture.

The ball, however, seemed to have a mind of its own. It met the scuffed wooden floor with a dull thud, bounced once, missed Marvin's waiting hands entirely, and rolled out of bounds, disappearing under the bleachers, a silent, anticlimactic conclusion to my attempt at connection. Marvin simply watched it go, his expression as unreadable as ever. The puzzle, it seemed, had just gained another piece, and I was no closer to solving it.

Returning to our unit was usually a ritual of fading into our respective roles. But that evening, our descent was interrupted. Standing directly in front of our door, silhouetted against the dim corridor light, was a man I didn't recognize. He was broad-shouldered, his uniform crisp despite the late hour, and an air of entitled impatience radiated from him.

He held up a hand, palm out, as if expecting a salute or, more likely, a direct answer. "My cigarettes," he grunted, his voice gravelly. "Seen anyone with them?"

The question hung in the air, innocuous enough on the surface, but for Marvin, it was a trigger. He walked towards the door, his movements jerky, and froze. His eyes, usually darting and unfocused, widened, locking onto the man. The color drained from his face, leaving his freckled complexion stark against the shadows.

I felt a surge of protective instinct, a familiar response to Marvin's peculiar vulnerability. He was a puzzle, a collection of unconnected behaviors and anxieties that made him a constant source of bewilderment, but also, strangely, of concern.

"You won't see Marvin," I said, my voice deliberately calm, projecting a confidence I didn't entirely feel. "And you won't get any cigarettes from him." I let the words hang there, a deliberate severing of expectation. "Not now. Not ever."

Marvin, perhaps hearing the conviction in my tone, the unspoken alliance, finally found his voice. It was a reedy sound, but it held a new, unexpected firmness. "Don't steal cigarettes," he said, his gaze still fixed on the man, a small accusation in his statement. Then, without another word, he slipped past the man and into the unit, disappearing into the relative safety of our shared space.

The man scowled, a dark cloud settling over his features. It was a petty annoyance for him, I imagined, a minor obstacle. But I knew, with a certainty that surprised even me, that it was okay. The micro-aggression, the assertion of ownership, had been met.

I followed Marvin inside. The unit was a familiar chaos of patient needs. Marvin made his way to his own corner, where his roommate, Jerry, was already sprawled on his bed, a faint, perpetual smile playing on his lips. Jerry was another enigma, passive and seemingly oblivious to the usual mental health dramas.

Without any preamble, no segue, no attempt at normal conversation, Marvin turned to Jerry. His voice, now laced with a bizarre, almost accusatory innocence, stated, "Jerry's pinching my tits."

Jerry's smile widened fractionally. He didn't deny it. He didn't even shift.

I'd learned to navigate these abrupt shifts in Marvin's reality. I looked at Jerry, my gaze steady. "Jerry, are you pinching Marvin's tits?"

"Yea," Jerry confirmed, his smile unwavering, entirely unperturbed.

"Don't do it anymore," I said, my tone firm but not aggressive. It was a directive, a simple instruction to halt an unwanted physical interaction.

Jerry, still smiling, nodded. "Okay."

And that was it. They walked away, Marvin a small, bewildered phantom, Jerry a placid shadow. They disappeared into the shared space, their peculiar interaction resolved with an almost absurd simplicity.

Marvin remained a mystery, a walking, talking Rorschach test. But that, I'd come to understand, was the point. My role wasn't to solve him, not entirely. It was about pattern recognition – identifying the strange rhythms of his behavior, the unexpected disruptions – and then, when necessary, pattern disruption. To nudge the edges of his world, to introduce a new variable, and to observe the ripple. And sometimes, like that day, to simply stand between him and a scowling man demanding cigarettes.

# Leonard

Leonard adjusted the knot of his crimson tie, the silk a cool whisper against his skin. He smoothed down the lapels of his navy blazer, a garment that always felt as if it had been sculpted for his frame. His slacks, a crisp charcoal grey, draped perfectly, creating a silhouette that spoke of deliberate attention and a subtle, inherent order. He surveyed his reflection in the hallway mirror, not with vanity, but with a quiet affirmation. The ensemble wasn't an affectation; it was a uniform, a declaration.

When he walked into my office, I was taken aback. Perhaps it was just the way his presence seemed to absorb the ambient noise. He didn't stride, but rather moved with a measured, almost deliberate gait, his shoulders held square, his chin held high enough to convey a considered perspective without tipping into arrogance. His gaze, when it swept across the faces of his family gathered for Sunday dinner, held a steady, intelligent gleam.

"So, Leonard, I understand you attended law school at Harvard. Quite impressive."

He didn't fidget or offer a vague, dismissive response. Instead, he offered a small, knowing smile, the kind that suggested he was privy to truths others hadn't yet grasped. He sat in the chair next to my desk, placing his hands, long-fingered and steady, on the polished wood.

"Yes," he said, his voice a smooth baritone, devoid of any youthful uncertainty. He paused, letting the weight of his statement settle. "In fact," he continued, his eyes meeting mine with an unwavering sincerity, "I've just finished my first year of law school."

The words landed with a quiet authority. There was no need for embellishment, no need to explain the late nights, the dense textbooks, the dizzying Socratic method. The way Leonard dressed, the way he carried himself – with that inherent sense of importance, that quiet confidence that radiated from him like a subtle perfume – it all simply fit. It was the unspoken, irrefutable evidence of his accomplishment, a testament to the rigor and dedication he had invested. No one in the room doubted him for a second. It was, for Leonard, the only way it could be.

The sterile scent of antiseptic and old linoleum clung to the air in Manteno State Hospital, a pervasive odor that promised neither rest nor relaxation. Sunlight, diluted by the thick panes of glass in my office, cast weak, institutional shadows.

"So, what brings you here, Leonard?"

Leonard's head snapped up, his eyes, though a little bloodshot, held an intense, almost frantic intelligence. "Rest. Relaxation." He recited the words with a practiced cadence, as if delivering them in a courtroom. "Law school is demanding. It puts a lot of pressure on a man. Especially Harvard."

He paused, taking a shallow breath, then plunged into a detailed explanation, his voice rising in pitch and tempo with each clause. "To achieve their pedagogical goals, Harvard Law School faculty use a variety of teaching methods in their classrooms. Students should be prepared for the fact that some of their faculty will use variations on the Socratic Method in the classroom for part or all of their class. This means faculty will ask students to be prepared to answer questions through one of or a combination of real-time questioning (e.g., cold calls where students are called on to answer questions without prior notice or warm calls where they are given some prior notice), panel systems, group deliberation and reporting back, among other modes of eliciting student participation. All students should be prepared to participate in the method of instruction a faculty member has designed for the course."

He finished, exhaling sharply, his chest heaving slightly. His gaze drifted past me, unfocused for a moment, before snapping back to her face. It was in this slight pause, this fleeting moment of vulnerability, that he added, almost as an afterthought, his voice barely a whisper against the lingering echo of his passionate recitation: "And I might be depressed."

I watched him, pen poised over her a notepad. I'd heard many explanations in this room, but few so meticulously delivered, so academically precise, yet so utterly devoid of personal emotion until that final, stark admission. It was as if he had built an elaborate legal brief for his own breakdown, citing the very methods that had perhaps chipped away at his sanity.

I nodded slowly. "I see. The Socratic method can be quite challenging." I kept my voice neutral, inviting him to elaborate on the feelings behind the facts.

Leonard's eyes narrowed slightly, as though he was assessing her statement for any potential weaknesses. "Challenging is an understatement. It's an intellectual gauntlet. Professor Thorne, for instance. He has a predilection for the 'cold call.'

Imagine, hundreds of pages of intricate legal theory, precedent upon precedent, and suddenly, he fixes you with that stare, that predatory gleam in his eye, and asks, 'Leonard, what is the ratio decidendi in Hadley v. Baxendale and how does it apply to the present case, assuming we are dealing with a breach of contract involving a defective cotton mill shaft?' One must not merely know the answer; one must present it, articulate it, defend it against his relentless cross-examination, all while your peers, your future rivals, dissect your every word."

He ran a hand through his already disheveled hair, a tremor in his fingers. "I began to anticipate them. To obsess. I'd read, reread, outlined until my vision blurred. I'd wake in a cold sweat, rehearsing answers to questions that hadn't even been asked yet. The library became a battleground. My dorm room, a solitary confinement cell for the intellectually damned."

The "rest and relaxation" now seemed a tragically ironic euphemism. I understood. The pressure hadn't merely been demanding; it had been crushing. The brilliance that allowed him to articulate the intricacies of Harvard's pedagogy had also been the very engine driving his descent. He hadn't just learned the law; he had become utterly consumed by it, until the lines between his identity and his academic performance blurred, then shattered.

"And the depression, Leonard?" I prompted gently. "How does that manifest?"

He looked at his hands, then away. "Manifest?" The word seemed to trip him. "A lack of... vigor. Anhedonia. A persistent feeling of... inadequacy. Despite the hours, the preparation. I couldn't sleep. Or I'd sleep too much. Food... it became an inconvenience. The world, the vibrant, competitive world I wanted to conquer, started to look rather... grey. As if all the colors had been drained."

He paused, a flicker of something raw and exposed in his eyes. "I just... stopped being able to function. My professors suggested... a sabbatical. My parents arranged... this." His gaze swept around the sparse room, taking in the muted tones, the secured window. "They preferred the term 'wellness retreat.' But I suppose... this is Manteno."

He finally looked at me and the intellectual armor he'd worn began to crack, revealing the exhausted, frightened young man underneath. The meticulous lawyer, arguing his case for admission, was gone. Only Leonard, the student who had lost himself in the pursuit of perfection, remained. And in his eyes, I saw not just the shadow of Harvard, but the deep, weary ache of a soul in need of true rest, far beyond the confines of any library or lecture hall.

I tapped a pen against the crisp white file in front of him, his gaze sharp and unwavering as it met Leonard's. The room was sterile, silent save for the hum of the ventilation system, a stark contrast to the vivid landscape Leonard's mind had just conjured.

"Let's finish up, Leonard. Just a few minor questions. Are you married? Or have you been married?"

Leonard, a man whose tailored tweed jacket seemed perpetually on the verge of shedding the dust of distant lands, leaned back in his chair. A faint, almost wistful smile touched his lips, crinkling the corners of eyes that had seen too much, or perhaps, just enough.

"I was married once. In Africa. By a witch doctor. It sounds strange, but it's true. A powerful woman, actually, a shaman of the N'gala tribe. We called her Mama Aziza." He paused, letting the words hang in the air, watching Me for a reaction. O merely jotted a note, his expression unreadable.

"But," Leonard continued, a sigh escaping him, "the tribe didn't accept me, not truly. And so the marriage was... cancelled. I don't remember the exact word they used for it, but it was thorough."

I finally looked up, my professional facade cracking just slightly to reveal a flicker of something akin to incredulity. "A witch doctor. In Africa. And the tribe didn't accept you. Can you elaborate, Leonard?"

Leonard's smile broadened, this time with a hint of genuine amusement. "Of course. This was... oh, fifteen years ago. I was embedded with a research team, studying rare medicinal plants in a particularly remote corner of the Congo basin. We'd pushed deeper than most, into lands largely untouched by modern influence. That's where I met Nomi. Her father was the elder, a man of immense wisdom, and Mama Aziza was their spiritual guide, their healer, their conduit to the ancestors."

He leaned forward, as if sharing a secret. "Nomi was remarkable. Fierce, intelligent, with eyes that saw into your very soul. She spent her days in the jungle, not just identifying plants, but communing with them. We fell in love, or what passed for it in that intense, isolated world. It was a whirlwind, driven by survival, by shared wonder, by the sheer, unadulterated passion of two souls finding each other against all odds."

"A whirlwind. Followed by a witch doctor wedding."

"Precisely," Leonard affirmed, unperturbed. "It wasn't a legal ceremony, not in any Western sense. It was a binding, a sacred union under the Banyan tree, witnessed by the spirits and the entire tribe. Mama Aziza wove our essences together with herbs, with chants, with the blood of a sacrificed goat. I wore a tribal loincloth, Nomi was adorned with flowers and paint. It was the most profound commitment of my life."

He paused, his gaze drifting to the sterile wall, seeing not plaster but dense jungle foliage. "For a while, it was idyllic. I learned their language, their customs. I hunted with the men, gathered with the women. I truly believed I was one of them, or at least, on my way to becoming so. But... I was always an outsider. My scientific mind, my need to quantify, to understand in a logical framework, it clashed with their intuitive, ancestral worldview. I couldn't fully believe in the spirits that spoke through Mama Aziza, not in the way they demanded. I couldn't see the world through their eyes, not completely. I tried. God, I truly did."

"And so, the rejection?" I prompted, sensing the pivot.

"Yes. A gradual cooling, a subtle distancing. Little slights at first, then more overt. They saw that my heart, though full of love for Nomi, was still rooted elsewhere. I lacked the necessary... conviction. The elders decided I wasn't truly married to the tribe, only to Nomi, and in their world, those were inseparable. A foreign root cannot nourish the same soil as a native one, they said."

Leonard's voice softened. "The 'cancellation' was even more elaborate than the wedding. A reverse ritual. Not a divorce, not a breaking of vows, but an un-binding. Mama Aziza called it 'The Un-rooting.' She said my essence, though momentarily intertwined, had failed to truly integrate with the soil of their ancestors. My spirit was to be returned to its original vessel, free to wander, unencumbered by the sacred ties I couldn't fully honor."

"And Nomi?" I asked, a rare note of genuine curiosity in his voice.

"Nomi understood. She was sad, heartbroken even, but she knew. She belonged to the tribe, to the spirits of the jungle. She couldn't leave, and I couldn't stay, not as a husband, not as a true member. The Un-rooting was painful, more spiritual than physical, a sense of having a part of yourself gently, but firmly, extracted. It left a hollow space."

Leonard met my gaze directly, his smile now gone, replaced by a quiet sincerity. "The word, the one I couldn't remember? It was 'Wavuaji.' It translates roughly to 'The Severance of the Deep Root.' And it meant I was un-married, yes, but also utterly un-belonged. I left a few weeks later. And I haven't been back."

I scribbled a final note, the pen scratching loud in the silence. I set down my notepad, the sound sharp and definitive. "Remarkable, Leonard. Truly remarkable. Thank you for your candor. Why don't you rest up while you're here?"

Leonard nodded, rising from his chair. As he walked towards the door, he couldn't help but wonder if his "un-rooted" past made him more, or less, suitable for whatever clandestine operation I represented. He left the sterile room, carrying the ghost of a Banyan tree and the echo of a forgotten tribal word, out into a world that often failed to understand the profound, inexplicable bonds he had once known.

Leonard was, to put it mildly, fascinating. His narrative was a tapestry woven with threads of the fantastical. He'd regaled me with tales of his elite education, his successful career, and then, the pièce de résistance: his marriage. Not just any marriage, mind you, but one conducted by a witch doctor in some exotic locale I couldn't quite place. I'd leaned in, scribbling feverishly, a small, unprofessional smile playing on my lips. This was going to be the highlight of the meeting, a moment of shared amusement amongst us jaded professionals. Leonard, with his grand pronouncements and peculiar beliefs, was a welcome deviation from the usual.

As I approached the conference room, ready to present my findings, a tiny, nagging voice of protocol nudged me. It was standard practice to touch base with the patient's family if possible. Leonard's sister, who lived with him, had provided the initial contact information. A quick call wouldn't hurt, I'd reasoned, and might even add a touch of color to my report.

I found her number and dialed. She answered with a warm, welcoming tone that immediately put me at ease. "Ms. Henderson? This is Brian from Manteno. I'm calling about your brother, Leonard."

"Oh, hello. How is he doing?" Her voice was gentle, tinged with that familiar familial worry.

"He's settling in. We've had our initial interview, and I wanted to clarify a few points with you before our team meeting this afternoon." I took a deep breath, ready to launch into Leonard's latest pronouncements. "Now, I understand Leonard mentioned he's attending Harvard Law School..."

There was a beat of silence on the other end, not an awkward silence, but one filled with an audible, almost musical, bemusement. "He said that?" Her voice was laced with a gentle disbelieving chuckle. "Bless his heart. He never went to law school. He barely finished high school."

My smile faltered. The hum of the fluorescent lights seemed to ratchet up a notch. "Oh," I managed, feeling a prickle of heat crawl up my neck. "Uh... so, he made that up?"

"No," she replied, her tone softening, "it's one of his delusions."

The words hung in the air. Delusion. The clinical term, so stark against the backdrop of Leonard's vibrant, if fabricated, life. I felt a wave of foolishness wash over me. How had I been so ready to accept such a grandiose claim without a flicker of doubt? My professional detachment had evaporated, replaced by a gullible eagerness for a good story. I pressed on, trying to salvage some semblance of my initial assessment. "Makes sense. Clearly, he has several delusions. This whole married by a witch doctor..." I trailed off, expecting her to confirm, perhaps with a weary sigh, the absurdity of it all.

Another pause. This one was different. It was a pregnant pause, heavy with unspoken implications.

"He was," she said, her voice steady, cutting through my assumptions like a sharp knife. "That part is true."

My mind reeled. "What?" The word was barely a whisper.

"He was married by a witch doctor," she repeated, a touch of something I couldn't quite identify – pride? Nostalgia? – entering her voice. "He visited Africa a few years back, and when he came home, he was married to an African woman. I can even send you the documents if you would like."

The hum of the lights faded completely, replaced by a roaring in my ears. Documents. A witch doctor. Africa. The neat, predictable narrative I had constructed for Leonard, the one I was preparing to present as a cautionary tale of delusion and fantasy, had just been rewritten by reality, in a way I could never have anticipated.

"Please," I managed, my voice catching. "Please, send them." The meeting was about to start, but my agenda had just been irrevocably altered. Leonard wasn't just a case of delusions; he was a man with a truth that was stranger, and far more compelling, than any fiction I had imagined. And I, the seasoned professional, had been utterly, wonderfully, outmaneuvered.

The air in the conference room at Manteno was thick with a familiar blend of exhaustion and quiet desperation. Fluorescent lights hummed overhead, casting a sterile glow on the circle of weary faces. I slipped in a few minutes late, my apology a mere murmur as I juggled my phone. I'd been on the line with Leonard's sister, a woman whose voice, even through the static, had carried the weight of years of worry.

As I looked around, seeing the slumped shoulders and the carefully neutral expressions, a sudden, fierce protectiveness surged through me. These were the people who had to make the tough calls, the ones who sifted through the fragments of shattered lives to find a path forward. And in this moment, I decided, they wouldn't be the only ones bearing the full burden of Leonard's story. I wouldn't let them be the only ones to see the complete, unvarnished truth of him.

So, I began to relay my conversation with his sister. I spoke of Leonard's recent agitation, his increasingly erratic behavior. Then, I leaned in, my voice steady, and said, "He told his sister he's been diligently studying for the bar exam. He believes he's preparing to practice law."

A subtle shift occurred in the room. A few heads tilted, a flicker of curiosity in previously deadened eyes. But no one flinched when I continued, adding, "Specifically, he's aiming for Harvard Law School."

There it was. The silence that followed was not one of disbelief, but of a strange, almost respectful acknowledgment of a mind that soared, even if in its isolation. It was the kind of silence that admitted the possibility, however remote, that this man, in his own reality, might just be capable of such an ambition. Years of dealing with patients had taught me that the human mind could construct elaborate tapestries of thought, and Leonard's was clearly a masterpiece of intricate detail.

Then, I delivered the sentence that would break the spell. "And his sister mentioned," I said, my gaze sweeping across the faces, "that he claimed to have been married by a witch doctor."

The dam broke. A ripple of laughter, hesitant at first, then growing in volume and heartiness, swept through the room. It wasn't cruel, not truly. It was the sound of release, the shared recognition of the absurdities that often accompanied profound struggles. It was the sound of a conclusion being reached, a diagnosis solidifying.

In that wave of laughter, the last vestiges of doubt, of the desperate hope that maybe, just maybe, he was still tethered to a more conventional reality, evaporated. In that moment, surrounded by the echoes of their mirth, it became undeniably clear to everyone in that room: Leonard, in his brilliant, peculiar, and deeply troubling way, definitely needed help.

The fluorescent lights of the conference room hummed, a familiar, sterile drone that usually faded into the background of our weekly treatment team meetings. Today, however, it felt amplified, a stark accompaniment to the silence that had fallen after my pronouncement. I swallowed, the dryness in my throat a tangible echo of the tension in the room.

"Then," I continued, my voice a little steadier than I'd expected, "I stated, 'I checked with his sister. You know, verified Leonard's story. Guess what? He never attended Harvard. But he truly was married by a witch doctor.'"

The silence that followed was thick, almost suffocating. Each face around the table reflected a similar, almost palpable, reaction. Ed, director of the unit, leaned back in his chair, his customary stern expression softened by a flicker of something unreadable. The nurse, usually quick with a dry observation, just blinked, her pen hovering motionless over her notepad. Even the pragmatic psychiatrist, looked momentarily thrown, his brow furrowed in a way that suggested he was grappling with more than just clinical data.

It was the look of disbelief. The same one I'd seen flash across Leonard's face when he'd first confessed his fabricated Harvard past. The same one that now mirrored my own, a strange blend of disappointment and reluctant admiration. It was the feeling of, somehow, being cheated. Not in a malicious way, but in a way that robbed us of a narrative we'd begun to embrace. Leonard, the brilliant, disillusioned Harvard grad who'd ended up here. It was a story with a tragic arc, a certain romanticism even.

But the witch doctor? That was... unexpected. And the verification of it, the utter, unassailable truth of it, was somehow more unsettling than the lie that had preceded it. It was as if the carefully constructed edifice of Leonard's delusion had crumbled, only to reveal something far more bizarre, far more grounding in its strangeness.

And truly, after all that, as I sat there and absorbed their collective bewilderment, a new thought began to crystallize. It wasn't about the delusion itself, or the patient's capacity for fantasy. It was about the craft of it. The sheer audacity, the intricate layering, the meticulous precision with which Leonard had woven not just one, but two distinct realities.

He had presented us with a carefully curated falsehood, an alibi, a persona. He had, in his own way, managed our perceptions. When one thread of his story was pulled, and the lie of Harvard was exposed, he hadn't crumbled. He had pivoted, revealing a truth so outlandish, so culturally specific, that for a moment, it felt like another carefully constructed diversion. But then, the confirmation. The sister's hesitant nod, the faint, knowing smile that suggested this was just another facet of her brother, the man who'd always been a little... beyond.

It hit me then, with a clarity that cut through the professional detachment. Leonard's talent wasn't just in manifesting delusions. It was in the subtle art of persuasion, the almost legalistic dismantling of one narrative and the subsequent construction of another. He'd understood, on an instinctual level, how to present evidence, how to gauge his audience, how to anticipate our skepticism.

And in that moment, watching the team process the bizarre truth of Leonard's marriage, I began to think that Leonard's talent to extract a delusion so layered and so precise, would make a great attorney. He wouldn't just represent a client; he'd reconstruct reality itself, brick by unbelievable brick, until the truth, or a version of it, was undeniable. And I, having witnessed his masterful performance, could only offer a silent, stunned applause.

---

The history of Manteno, the colossal complex of brick and discipline, is recorded meticulously in state archives, bound volumes full of diagnoses, admission dates, and expenditure reports. It is a history of the institution.

But within those walls, and across the hundreds of acres where the patients were permitted to walk their prescribed paths, lived the history of the soul. This documented history is cold and wide; the human history is narrow, burning, and utterly unique.

This is just a small sample of the people who inhabited that sprawling geography of vulnerability.

**Elias: The Cartographer of Light**

Elias had been at Manteno since 1938. His official record spoke of catatonic schizophrenia and the quiet, immovable nature of his presence. Staff often referred to him as "The Statue in the Solarium."

But Elias was not still; he was tracking.

His joy was the sun. Every morning, he would find the exact spot in the sun parlor where the light hit the floor tiles just so, illuminating the tiny granules of red aggregate embedded in the cement. He moved his chair only fractionally throughout the day, following the progress of the heat and the brightness as if it were a migratory bird he was charting.

Elias's unique personality was defined by his patience. He could wait three hours for a sparrow to land on the outer windowsill, and when it did, he would emit a low, guttural sigh of satisfaction—a sound that, to the untrained ear, sounded like discomfort, but was, in truth, profound appreciation.

His fear, however, was metallic and absolute: the sound of the key turning in the lock of the dayroom door. Elias knew that sound meant the loss of freedom, the imposition of the night, or, worse, the arrival of the attendants for a "treatment." When the key rattled, Elias's hands, resting placidly on his lap, would clench into such tight fists that his knuckles flared white, radiating silent, decades-old terror through his frail body. He knew the sun parlor would always bring the light back, but the keys were the permanent assurance of the walls.

**Clara: The Weaver of Worlds**

Clara arrived in the early 1950s, a girl of seventeen who possessed a mind too bright and fast for the slow, rigid world outside. Her file cited delusional grandiosity and manic episodes. To the world, she was a flight risk; to the few who watched her close enough, she was an architect.

Clara's great joy was her maps.

She carried scraps of paper—margins torn from old newspapers, brown wrapping paper filched from the kitchen, the backs of blank medical forms. Using charcoal stolen from the boiler room, or sometimes just chewed ballpoint pens, she created elaborate, impossible geographies.

These weren't maps of Manteno. These were maps of Aethel, the land where the gravity was optional, and Veridian, the city built entirely of spun glass, where the inhabitants communicated only by the shifting colors of light. Her personality was in the details: she drew tiny harbors where the boats were shaped like swans, and mountains that erupted with harmless, glittering steam.

The staff saw her frantic drawing as compulsive behavior. But for Clara, the moment the pen touched the paper, the walls of the brick facility dissolved. She was a ruler, a sovereign of shimmering dust and infinite possibility.

Her fear was not being locked up, but being forgotten. Her deepest, most debilitating fear was that the vibrant, complex cities she drew were the only thing keeping her memory of her mother's voice alive.

If the maps stopped, the voice—light and clear, singing old Irish lullabies—would fade into the institutional silence. She drew not for escape, but for preservation.

**Nurse Evelyn: The Keeper of Names**

Nurse Evelyn worked the night shift in Ward B, the ward known for its "difficult" cases. She was a woman hardened by years of procedure, but softened by an empathy the official reports never acknowledged. She was tasked with recording symptoms. She recorded something else entirely.

Evelyn understood that the documented history was a lie of omission.

For her, the humanity lay in the rituals. She knew that Mr. Abernathy was not sleeping poorly, he was simply waiting every night for the 3:00 AM train whistle from the distant Kankakee line, believing it was the signal for his long-deceased wife to finally arrive.

She knew Miss Davies's rage was not a spontaneous outburst, but a reaction to the smell of lemon disinfectant, which reminded her of the orphanage where she was abandoned.

Evelyn's unique task was to catalog their humanity when the documents insisted they had none. She kept a small, unauthorized notebook—a private, contraband history—tucked into her uniform pocket.

Elias's Joy: Today, the sun was a perfect circle on the floor. He smiled with his eyes.

Clara's Fear: Her hand trembled today. Gave her a cup of warm tea and told her Veridian needs strong foundations. She calmed immediately.

Evelyn knew that Manteno was a place built to contain chaos, but the people inside were not chaos. They were simply people whose inner lives were too grand, too fragile, or too wounded to operate by common consensus.

Over the course of decades, Manteno gathered these individuals in their thousands. The official account stands as a necessary record of an era—the architecture, the policies, the unfortunate treatments.

But the breathing, felt history is in the small moments: the weight of Elias's fear when the latch clicked home; the triumphant, secret beauty of Clara's nonexistent continents; and the quiet, persistent diligence of Nurse Evelyn, who ensured that the small sample of humanity living inside those massive walls would not be lost to the cold indifference of the archive. They were more than symptoms. They were a tapestry of unique joys and enduring fears, woven silently into the brutal, historic brickwork of Manteno.

# A Broader View

A cognitive psychologist whose career had been meticulously dedicated to dissecting the intricate mechanisms of epistemic rigidity, the stubborn, often pathological, resistance to revising one's beliefs in the face of contradictory evidence, sat hunched in the cavernous, dimly lit expanse of his office. The sole illumination emanated from the cool, blue-white glow of his monitor, casting an almost spectral pallor over the towering, precarious stacks of clinical files that bristled on every available surface, their worn edges testament to countless shattered realities. The air was thick with the faint, comforting scent of old paper and the quiet hum of his high-powered workstation, a sound that had become an almost constant companion in his solitary nocturnal work.

His focus was currently riveted on the digital intake notes for Patient 78-B, a case that, even by his extensive experience, presented a vivid, almost theatrical, tableau of distorted perception. She was a woman, middle-aged and otherwise appearing lucid, who possessed an unshakeable, genuinely held conviction that the neighborhood's feline population, far from merely chasing mice, was actively receiving codified messages beamed directly into her home through her aging television aerial.

To her, these enigmatic broadcasts, she claimed, dictated the precise, fluctuating prices of global commodities, from crude oil futures to the value of platinum on the international market. She meticulously documented these alleged feline pronouncements, convinced she held the key to universal economic understanding. A burden that weighed heavily on her.

He sighed, a deep, weary exhalation that seemed to carry the weight of every illogical narrative he had ever encountered. He ran a hand, calloused from years of gripping pens and tracing thought patterns, through his already thinning, salt-and-pepper hair, his gaze momentarily drifting to the framed diplomas on the wall, symbols of a scientific certainty that felt increasingly distant.

He noted, almost instinctively, the standard markers of a fixed belief system: the complete lack of verifiable proof despite her voluminous "research" and diagrams; the intense, almost visceral emotional distress upon challenge, where even gentle questioning would trigger anxiety, anger, or profound sadness; and, most significantly, how this fantastical belief had become central to her identity structure, defining her purpose, her daily routines, and her understanding of the world.

The diagnostic system, a meticulously constructed edifice of psychiatric understanding, had a ready-made category for such phenomena: delusion. It was, by definition, a "fixed, false belief that is contrary to reality testing," an unyielding conviction that persisted despite irrefutable evidence to the contrary and was not culturally normative. Patient 78-B fit the criteria perfectly, a textbook example of a mind fractured from consensus reality.

But lately, something profound was shifting within him. The sturdy, well-defined walls of his specialty felt thin, almost permeable, no longer offering the reassuring solidity of a contained field of study.

His meticulously observed pathologies, once clear and distinct, were beginning to blur at the edges, dissolving into a larger, more unsettling pattern. His work, once a precise dissection of individual cognitive malfunction, felt less like studying a discrete, unfortunate pathology and more like examining the micro-scale expression of a phenomenon that, in varying degrees of intensity and subject matter, dominated the entire human landscape.

He was no longer just seeing mental illness; he was seeing the foundational mechanism of belief itself, stripped bare and amplified, reflected disturbingly in the wider world beyond his office walls.

He wasn't suggesting the general public was clinically ill. Rather, he was arguing that the symptoms we isolate, medicate, and label as pathology in the individual are the exact mechanisms relied upon by the largest, most pervasive belief systems of modern society. The only difference between Patient 78-B and the millions of people adhering rigidly to an unprovable ideology, he concluded, was the scale of consensus.

He called it the "Sanctuary of Shared Myth."

**The Architecture of Unverifiable Belief**

When we examine the rigid adherence to beliefs that lack empirical evidence, we find three key characteristics that define both clinical delusion and large-scale societal adherence.

**1. Rigidity Despite Contradictory Evidence**

In the clinic, this manifests as the patient's inability to integrate data that conflicts with their core narrative. A patient who believes they are immune to gravity will dismiss the fact that they fall when they jump, explaining it away with increasingly complex, personalized rationalizations (e.g., "The floor is magnetically compensating for my true state").

This comprehensive adherence to ideologically rigid political beliefs marks a profound shift in the function of modern democracy, transitioning the political sphere from a marketplace of policy ideas to a battleground of existential, often fabricated, truths. This phenomenon is characterized by an epistemological crisis where foundational reality is supplanted by emotionally validating, conspiratorial narratives.

**2. The Discarding of Empirical Reality**

The source of these rigid political viewpoints is not a rational analysis of policy effectiveness, tax rates, or infrastructure planning, but rather a deeply personalized investment in grand, often paranoiac, conspiratorial narratives. Millions of individuals across the globe have adopted political truths that rely entirely on conjecture and are impervious to conventional empirical challenge. These beliefs persist long after they have been systematically invalidated by established methodologies: rigorous investigative bodies, statistical analysis by dedicated data scientists, verified public records, and formalized public hearings.

A belief that a global cabal controls weather patterns may persist even after satellite data, climate models, and meteorological records contradict it.

The adherence to these narratives transcends simple disagreement; it represents a commitment to an alternative reality.

Despite meticulous, often bipartisan, recounts, post-election audits, judicial reviews that failed in dozens of courts due to lack of evidence, and the consistent testimony of non-partisan election officials, the belief in a massive institutional plot to manipulate election results remains firmly entrenched. For adherents, the absence of proof is simply interpreted as the perfection of the concealment, creating a logic where the transparency of the democratic process is proof of its corruption.

Equally pervasive are beliefs surrounding a global institutional plot to harm the population via medicine, often centered on vaccine efficacy or mandates. Claims suggesting government agencies (such as the CDC or FDA), alongside major pharmaceutical entities, are actively engaged in population control or deliberate poisoning are thoroughly disproven by comprehensive scientific literature, peer-reviewed studies, and widespread global health data. Yet, the narrative persists, fueled by an identity-defining mistrust of experts, academics, and regulatory infrastructure.

### 3. The Mechanism of Cognitive Insulation: The Self-Sealing Argument

The defining characteristic of this ideological adherence is its self-sealing nature—the ability to interpret contradictory evidence not as a refutation, but as definitive proof of the conspiracy itself.

Just as the hypothetical patient attempts to explain away gravity by insisting that a secret, undetectable force must be lifting them, the devoted ideological adherent employs a sophisticated psychological defense mechanism to explain away verifiable facts.

When an independent body (e.g., an audit firm, a federal judge, or a scientific journal) produces data that contradicts the core conspiracy theory, that data is instantly recast through a conspiratorial lens.

**The Source is Compromised**: The investigators who produced the contradictory data (the auditors, the scientists, the journalists) are immediately assumed to be compromised. They are deemed financially incentivized, blackmailed, or, most commonly, part of the "deep state" apparatus they were tasked to investigate.

**The Evidence is Fabricated**: The finding itself is viewed as manufactured cover-up. For example, the claim—"The audit only found that the election was legitimate because the deep state paid them off to suppress the real findings"—transforms the institution tasked with seeking the truth into the chief antagonist of the narrative.

**Reinforcement of Paranoia**: This process serves to reinforce the initial paranoia. Every effort to debunk the conspiracy becomes evidence of how powerful and far-reaching the conspiracy truly is, creating a closed loop of belief that becomes impenetrable to external, objective reality.

### 4. The Resulting Epistemological Crisis

This widespread reliance on self-sealing narratives fundamentally undermines the shared epistemic foundation necessary for a functioning democracy. When facts are relative and institutional authority is intrinsically suspect, the populace loses the ability to distinguish between credible, verified information and malicious conjecture. The resulting crisis is not merely political; it is a breakdown in the common understanding of reality, making collective decision-making, policy consensus, and trust in the rule of law virtually impossible.

Because this belief is shared by millions, it is not labeled delusional. It is labeled "loyalty" or "alternative truth." The individual finds validation in the sheer volume of co-believers, reinforcing the rigidity.

### 5. Emotional Distress and Identity Fusion

A defining characteristic of clinical delusion is the intensity of the emotional reaction when the belief is questioned. Challenge the patient's delusion, and you trigger panic, rage, or deep personal threat. This is because the delusion is not just a belief; it is the keystone of their self-identity and their framework for understanding reality.

---

For billions across the globe, religious faith transcends mere affiliation; it forms the irreducible, foundational core of their very identity. It is the comprehensive narrative framework that explains their origins (their perceived past), dictates their behavior in the present, and guarantees their destiny (their projected future). This deep integration supplies an unequivocal moral compass, an absolute cosmology, and an ultimate, non-negotiable moral purpose.

These defining convictions often include the absolute certainty of highly specific, detailed visions of the afterlife—a promised paradise or a threatened damnation—or the unwavering belief in specific historical divine interventions, miraculous events, and sacred texts delivered by definitive decree. Crucially, these tenets exist entirely outside the domain of empirical methodology; they are assertions a priori, none of which can be scientifically verified or submitted to repeatable experimental scrutiny.

When these core tenets are challenged—when an adversary demands empirical proof of a soul's migration, the mechanics of resurrection, or the literal recording of a divine command—the resulting encounter is rarely a detached, academic debate. The response is almost universally visceral, immediate, and profoundly defensive, manifesting as sharp anger, preemptive dismissal, searing moral outrage, and acute psychological distress. This is not merely a strong disagreement; it is a profound existential crisis playing out in real-time. The challenger is not engaging a mere scientific hypothesis or debating historical probability; they are attempting to dismantle the individual's entire structure of meaning, their existential anchor, and their very reason for being.

Furthermore, when such a belief defines the shared reality of five million people (or five hundred million), the resulting collective outrage is rapidly reinterpreted within the group dynamic. Individual psychological distress and defensive counter-attack are recast as "moral fortitude," "righteous anger," or the valorous act of "defending sacred ground," effectively masking the underlying stress reaction to an identity-threatening challenge.

This collective consensus allows the group to execute the final, strategic move: granting the belief absolute immunity from rational or empirical scrutiny by explicitly designating it "faith"—a higher form of knowledge that, by definition, requires belief without evidence. This deliberate insulation mechanism ensures the foundational structure remains inviolable, placing the core identity beyond the reach of external logic.

For a staggering number of people—counted in the billions—religious faith is far more than a simple label on a questionnaire or an occasional Sunday-morning habit. It is the irreducible and foundational core of who they are. In the same way that a nation's constitution defines the limits and liberties of its citizens, faith supplies the ultimate charter for the individual. It does not merely sit alongside other aspects of self-definition (occupation, ethnicity, political affiliation); it constitutes the very scaffolding on which all other self-descriptions are erected.

Faith provides a comprehensive narrative framework that stretches across three temporal dimensions.

**Origins (the perceived past):** A story of creation, a mythic lineage, or a divine election that tells the believer where they come from. "I am a child of Abraham, chosen by God from the very beginning of history."

**Present conduct (the lived moment)**: Explicit prescriptions for how to think, speak, eat, dress, work, and relate to others. "The Ten Commandments dictate my daily decisions; prayer is the rhythm of my day."

**Future destiny (the projected future)**: A promise of an after-life, a final judgment, or an eschatological fulfilment that gives purpose to every present action. "My soul will be welcomed into Paradise if I keep the faith; otherwise it faces eternal separation."

Because the story is totalizing, every experience—joyful, tragic, mundane, or extraordinary—is interpreted through its lens. A birth, a death, a natural disaster, or a personal success is not merely a random event; it is a sign, a test, or a fulfillment of a divine script.

The ethical code that emerges from scripture, prophetic tradition, or revelation is treated as absolute and non-negotiable. It is not a set of cultural conventions open to revision; rather, it is the law of the universe as inscribed by a transcendent authority. Consequently, moral judgments are experienced as self-evident truths: "lying is wrong because it violates God's command, not because society says so."

Faith supplies an absolute cosmology—an all-encompassing account of how the world and the multiverse came into being, why suffering exists, and what ultimate reality looks like. This cosmology is often articulated in creation myths, prophetic visions, or theological treatises that stand outside the realm of scientific explanation.

The belief that life has a non-negotiable moral purpose—to serve, love, or worship the divine—provides an unshakable sense of meaning. The purpose is not contingent on personal ambition or societal recognition; it is prescribed by the divine order itself.

Most religious traditions augment the above framework with highly detailed visions of the after-life or concrete accounts of divine intervention. After-life scenarios – vivid descriptions of heaven as a garden of endless light, or hell as a furnace of unending torment, complete with hierarchies of angels and demons, rewards, and punishments for specific earthly deeds.

Miraculous events – narratives of prophets parting seas, saints healing the sick with a touch, or sacred texts being delivered through fire-borne tablets that no human could have authored.

These particulars are not peripheral embellishments; they are core data points that believers memorize, recite, and use as benchmarks for personal conduct. The certainty attached to them is often expressed in absolute terms: "I know for certain that after death I will be judged by God" or "The Qur'an was revealed verbatim to Muhammad by the Angel Gabriel."

Crucially, the propositions described above are *a priori*—they are asserted as true independently of any sensory observation or experimental verification. Their status is deliberately insulated from the empirical method:

**Non-falsifiability** – No laboratory can capture a soul's migration, nor can a physicist design an apparatus that records a divine command.

**Irreproducibility** – Miraculous events are singular, historically unique, and presented as once-in-history interventions, making them immune to repeatable testing.

**Transcendence of measurement** – Concepts such as "eternal bliss" or "divine will" are defined in metaphysical terms that elude quantification.

Because of this, believers and religious institutions often articulate a principle of "faith without evidence": the truth of these claims rests on trust rather than on proof.

When an interlocutor—whether a scientist, an atheist, or a skeptical insider—asks for empirical proof of these central claims, the encounter is rarely a calm, academic exchange. The response typically unfolds in a cascade of visceral, defensive reactions:

**Immediate Anger** – A surge of physiological arousal (increased heart rate, tightened muscles) that manifests as sharp, often uncontrollable anger.

**Preemptive Dismissal** – A reflexive labeling of the challenger as "ignorant," "hostile," or "heretical," which serves to discredit the source before the argument proceeds.

**Moral Outrage** – A feeling that the challenger is not only wrong but evil, because they appear to be attacking the very foundation of the believer's existence.

**Psychological Distress** – Anxiety, dread, or even panic, as the individual perceives a threat to their existential anchor—the sense that their life's meaning is being ripped away.

These reactions are not merely disagreements over facts; they constitute a full-blown existential crisis that occurs in real time. The mind interprets the question not as "Can we test the resurrection?" but as "*Are we being told that everything I believe, everything that gives my life purpose, is a lie?*"

When the belief in question is shared by millions (or even billions), the individual's defensive state is quickly reframed by the group's cultural narrative:

**Moral Fortitude** – The anger is presented as courage in the face of hostile secular forces.

**Righteous Anger** – The emotional fire is labeled "holy" and "justified," turning a personal feeling into a collective virtue.

**Defending Sacred Ground** – The act of speaking out becomes a mission to protect the community's sacred territory from contamination.

By recasting personal stress as collective heroism, the group creates a social environment where defensive counter-attacks are celebrated, not pathologized. This social reinforcement amplifies the emotional response and makes it more difficult for the individual to retreat into self-questioning.

Within this communal framework, a deliberate protective mechanism is enacted: the belief system is formally labeled as "faith." This label serves several strategic purposes:

Faith is declared a higher epistemic category, above reason, science, and empirical observation. By definition, anything categorized as faith requires belief without evidence; therefore, attempts at logical or scientific critique are deemed irrelevant or even sacrilegious. The core identity, is thereby placed beyond the reach of external logic—ritualized, sanctified, and immunized from empirical breach.

The statement holds a profound truth about the structure of modern medicine: Insurance companies and pharmaceutical manufacturers are the dominant architects and controlling nexus of healthcare delivery, serving as the ultimate arbiters of access, cost, and innovation, irrespective of how that care is initially financed.

This architecture—designed not by healers but by financiers—will be examined in the next chapter, where the choreography of access, denial, and profit is laid bare.

# GOVERNING POWERS OF MENTAL HEALTH TREATMENT

## The Insurance Companies: The Gatekeepers of Access

Insurance companies (or payers), whether they manage massive governmental programs (like Medicare Advantage or state Medicaid contracts) or private employer-sponsored plans, function as the primary gatekeepers between the patient, the provider, and the treatment. Their governance is rooted in financial optimization and risk management, which often supersedes clinical necessity.

**Prior Authorization and Utilization Review**: Insurers mandate that providers justify certain expensive procedures, specialty referrals, or diagnostic tests before they can be administered. This process imposes administrative friction, often delaying care and subtly discouraging providers from prescribing treatments deemed too costly or experimental.

**Tiered Formularies**: Insurance companies dictate which drugs they will cover and at what co-pay level. Their formulary committees negotiate aggressively with pharmaceutical companies, classifying drugs into tiers. This forces patients to often adopt cheaper, "preferred" alternatives (which benefit the insurer financially) even if their physician recommended a newer, potentially more effective, but non-preferred therapeutic.

**Network Restriction**: By establishing narrow provider networks, insurers control where patients can receive care. They steer patients toward systems that agree to lower reimbursement rates, effectively shaping the economic viability of hospitals and specialist groups.

In essence, insurers govern by controlling the flow of care, transforming the provider's clinical recommendation into a corporate decision about cost-effectiveness.

### The Pharmaceutical Companies: The Dictators of Price and Innovation

Pharmaceutical companies control the essential tools of modern medicine: the medications and therapeutics themselves. Their governance is established through patents, research investment, and unparalleled pricing power, which fundamentally dictates the baseline cost of treating virtually every illness.

**Unconstrained Pricing Power**: In many markets, particularly the United States, pharmaceutical pricing is detached from manufacturing costs or clinical benefits. Companies set prices based on "what the market will bear" (i.e., the perceived value to the patient and the solvency of the payer). This leads to exorbitant costs for vital drugs, especially high-cost specialty biologics and cancer treatments.

**Directing Research & Development**: Pharma companies prioritize research into conditions that promise the largest and most reliable financial return. While they are responsible for life-saving innovations, their profit imperative can lead to under-investment in rare diseases, low-income global health issues, or non-patentable public health solutions (like antibiotics).

**Patent Protection and Monopoly**: Through complex patent thickets and regulatory exclusivity, pharmaceutical firms maintain decades-long monopolies on key therapeutics. This stifles competition, ensures sustained high prices, and limits the ability of generic manufacturers to drive costs down.

Pharma companies govern by controlling the value of care, ensuring that any financial structure—whether public or private—must allocate significant resources to pay for their products.

### The Coalescing Force: A Dynamic of Interdependence

The true governing power lies in the strategic interdependence between these two corporate sectors. They operate in a continuous negotiation cycle:

**Pharma creates expensive products.**

Insurers must decide whether (and how much) to pay for them. They demand large rebates and volume discounts in exchange for placing the drug favorably on their formulary.

The rebates and costs are eventually passed back to the patient or the taxpayer through higher premiums or rising government healthcare expenditures.

This creates a system where maximizing financial returns—not maximizing public health—is the highest priority. The result is a healthcare landscape where the choice of therapeutics, the speed of access, and the overall affordability are ultimately decided in corporate boardrooms, rather than in the consulting room or the legislative chamber, already woven into the fabric of personal and collective life, becomes untouchable—any attack on it is automatically framed as an attack on the whole community.

The community can sanction strong, even coercive, responses (e.g., censorship, legal penalties, social ostracism) under the banner of protecting "faith." The result is an insulation mechanism that keeps the foundational structure of belief invulnerable to external logic, ensuring that the identity it supports remains beyond the reach of rational debate.

**The Therapist of Consensus**

The good doctor pushed back from his desk, the image of Patient 78-B's frantic, convinced eyes merging seamlessly with the images flashing on the news screen overhead—protesters railing against undeniable facts, politicians doubling down on falsified history.

The difference, he realized, was not in the psychological mechanism, but in the social validation.

The individual with a mental illness suffers an epistemic fracture—a break between their personal reality and the shared reality. They are isolated, and their system is deemed "maladaptive" because it fails to integrate with the 99% consensus.

But the millions who cling rigidly to political falsehoods, who defend unprovable religious details unto death, or who ignore measurable economic disaster to maintain an ideological purity, are not isolated. They are conformed.

Their symptoms—rigidity, defensiveness, certainty where proof is absent—are simply amplified by the collective. Society does not label these beliefs delusional; it labels them "worldviews."

And in this amplified state, the mental anguish that might drive a single person to therapy becomes the collective, driving force behind wars, polarization, and cultural stagnation.

"We diagnose the private symptom," the doctor muttered, clicking off his lamp. "But we celebrate the public one. We treat the solitary person who believes they are chosen by the sky, yet we build monuments to the millions who believe they are chosen by the heavens. The underlying psychology of conviction without proof remains identical. It is merely the scale of acceptance that determines whether we seek a cure or demand allegiance."

# The Institution

The true architecture of the institution, far from being a collection of simplistic, visible constructs like steel bars, reinforced glass panes, or the imposing concrete boundaries that traditionally define a physical perimeter, is in fact an intangible yet omnipresent structure. This contemporary form of confinement sheds the need for overt physical walls because its design is infinitely more insidious and effective: it exists entirely within the sophisticated mechanisms of systemic control and pervasive psychological conditioning.

This modern institution operates through an intricate web of systemic controls. These are the often-unseen laws, policies, bureaucratic procedures, economic imperatives, and social norms that subtly yet profoundly dictate the parameters of individual existence. It's the fine print in contracts, the debt cycles that bind individuals to specific work or lifestyles, the standardized educational pathways that channel ambition into predefined roles, the healthcare protocols that govern access and treatment, and the media narratives that shape collective understanding and belief. These systems create an invisible labyrinth, guiding choices, limiting possibilities, and establishing a default "normal" that, once internalized, becomes difficult to question or deviate from. The boundaries are not visible fences; they are the invisible lines enforced by the threat of economic precarity, social ostracization, or administrative punishment, creating a perpetual state of self-regulation.

Complementing and reinforcing these systemic layers is the equally potent force of psychological conditioning. This is the continuous, often subliminal process through which individuals are shaped to accept, endorse, and even champion the very systems that constrain them. It begins in early education, is reinforced by mass media, advertising, and popular culture, and is solidified by peer pressure and societal expectations. Through constant exposure, individuals are conditioned to desire specific consumer goods, aspire to certain career paths, adhere to particular social values, and fear non-conformity.

Critical thought can be subtly undermined, replaced by a preference for comfortable consensus. This conditioning fosters a subtle yet profound self-censorship and an internalized sense of obligation, where the individual becomes their own most effective guard. The "cells" are no longer physical rooms, but rather the narrow confines of prescribed thought, the fear of judgment, and the self-imposed limitations born from a lifetime of controlled inputs.

Thus, the true architecture of the institution is a complex, symbiotic relationship between external, pervasive systems and deeply internalized psychological frameworks. It's an everywhere-and-nowhere prison where the individual is often unaware of their incarceration, or, tragically, actively participates in maintaining their own confinement and that of others. Breaking free from this structure doesn't involve scaling walls, but rather a profound awakening to the invisible threads of control and the mental programming that defines one's perceived reality.

It is first and foremost built upon a substrate of shared beliefs—the insidious, quiet consensus, sometimes termed "therapeutic dogma," that governs acceptable behavior, diagnoses deviance, and enforces normalization. These beliefs are the ideological walls, allowing the institution to expand far beyond its physical address; they are the self-policing mechanisms that turn patients, staff, and even family members into complicit gatekeepers of conformity.

The second tier of its construction is not forged from iron and mortar, but from a far more insidious and deeply penetrating substance: chemical restraints. This represents the ultimate unseen pharmacological governance, a sophisticated system that replaces the overt clanking of visible chains and the stark reality of barred windows with the subtle tremor of altered neurochemistry. Here, control is not imposed upon the body from without, but meticulously orchestrated within the very fabric of an individual's consciousness and physiology through a precisely calibrated cocktail of psychoactive agents.

This is the calculated deployment, not of random medication, but of specific psychotropic drugs designed to achieve a singular, overarching objective: absolute, docile compliance. Sedatives are administered to dull the sharp edges of anxiety and agitation, inducing a compliant lethargy that saps the will to resist or even question. Mood stabilizers are employed to smooth out the tumultuous landscape of emotion, preventing not only the dangerous highs of defiance or mania but also the debilitating lows of despair that might fuel rebellion or profound introspection. Antipsychotics, beyond their primary use in suppressing delusions or hallucinations, often function to blunt the very capacity for independent thought or potent feeling, bringing with them a profound state of apathy and reduced initiative.

The cumulative effect is to flatten any dangerous peaks of emotion or resistance – be it anger, despair, or even revolutionary fervor – into a manageable, insipid plateau. This chemically enforces a state of profound stasis, not merely calm, but an almost anesthetized existence where volatility is neutralized and vibrant personality is flattened into predictable, unchallenging behavior. The institution's power, therefore, lies not in the crude imposition of physical confinement, but in its chilling ability to regulate an individual's most intimate internal experience.

It transcends mere external control, delving deep into the very substrate of consciousness, dampening volition, recalibrating perception, and silencing dissent before it can even form. A vibrant, perhaps defiant, personality is pathologized into a series of "symptoms" – agitation, grandiosity, non-compliance – which are then expertly managed, mitigated, and ultimately suppressed via the relentless rhythm of scheduled doses, transforming a volatile human spirit into controlled symptomatology, a perpetual, internal subjugation.

The ultimate structural support for this precarious, often inhumane ecosystem is the very apparatus designed to prevent its collapse: the crushing weight of bureaucratic barriers erected in the name of "help."

Finally, the entire edifice is buttressed by this dense, administrative friction, creating a paralyzing environment defined by sclerotic processes and procedural oppression. This is not mere inefficiency; it is a structural design where complexity acts as a strategic gatekeeper. The system demands the translation of urgent human suffering into sterile, encoded data via labyrinthine forms—documents that sprawl across multiple pages, requiring information that is often inaccessible or irrelevant to the immediate crisis. These forms are backed by arbitrary and constantly shifting budgetary restrictions, which are then enforced by layers of endless committees. These committees function primarily as mechanisms of risk mitigation and avoidance, perpetually shifting responsibility and delaying any definitive action.

Genuine outreach, promised in the institution's charter, is systematically transformed into a system of perpetual deference and denial. The 'help' becomes a distant, theoretical possibility, an oasis shimmering on the horizon, yet infinitely retreating. Access is endlessly deferred by petty, yet mandatory rituals: the required chase for triplicate signatures, each one representing another department, another layer of liability, and another week lost. This is followed by multi-week, invasive assessments designed less to understand the need and more to confirm the applicant's potential unworthiness or ineligibility. The critical necessity of referrals often proves the final, insurmountable hurdle, demanding prerequisite documents or appointments that are functionally impossible for the struggling, already marginalized individual to obtain.

In this chilling reality, the institution ceases to be a proactive conduit for support and becomes the friction itself. It embodies an overwhelming administrative inertia—a massive, energy-draining force that ensures those trapped within the system remain hopelessly stationary. The user is beaten down not by the absence of resources, but by the sheer, soul-crushing effort demanded simply to navigate the mandated protocols. Exhaustion is the system's primary output. The very struggle required to escape its cycles of mandated care guarantees that the desperate remain stationary, depleted by the overwhelming administrative gauntlet necessary just to secure the privilege of being marginally recognized.

# The Shift We Need

The path to authentic mental health treatment begins, first and foremost, at the recognition of the individual labeled as the "patient" not as a collection of symptoms or a static diagnosis, but fundamentally as a human being, a complex and intrinsic member of the human race.

This foundational recognition is the ethical and philosophical pivot upon which all genuine therapeutic progress rests. It demands that the healthcare professional move beyond the reductionist paradigm that often dominates clinical settings—where an individual is primarily seen as a manifestation of a pathology (e.g., "the Schizophrenic" or "the Borderline")—and instead acknowledges their inherent dignity, their full narrative, and their profound complexity.

To recognize the patient as a human being is to affirm their intrinsic worth, regardless of the severity or nature of their distress. It means understanding that mental suffering is often an intensely human response to life's traumas, biological predispositions, and environmental stressors, not merely a deficiency to be eradicated. This recognition entails seeing:

**Context and History**: They possess a unique life story, a network of relationships, cultural background, economic realities, and prior experiences that shape their current state. Their identity is not defined by their illness but merely informed by it.

**Agency and Autonomy**: They retain the capacity for self-determination, decision-making, and contribution, even when severely impaired. Treatment must prioritize respecting their autonomy, fostering empowerment, and collaborating actively in the recovery plan, rather than dictating solutions.

**Shared Vulnerability**: The professional must acknowledge the common ground of human fragility. By seeing the shared membership in the human race, the rigid hierarchy between the 'healer' and the 'afflicted' diminishes, fostering an essential environment of empathy, trust, and non-judgment.

When the patient is humanized, the therapeutic model fundamentally shifts:

**From Management to Partnership**: Treatment ceases to be merely the management of symptoms (via medication or restrictive behavioral control) and transforms into a collaborative journey toward recovery, growth, and the rediscovery of meaning.

**From Deficit-Focus to Strength-Focus**: Clinicians are compelled to look beyond the deficiencies listed in diagnostic criteria and actively seek out the individual's existing strengths, resilience, hopes, and untapped potential.

**Holistic and Ethical Care**: Recognition of the patient as a whole person necessitates a holistic approach that integrates biological factors with psychological, social, cultural, and spiritual components of well-being. This ethical groundwork ensures that interventions are applied in service of the individual's flourishing, rather than merely fitting the individual into a standardized protocol.

Ultimately, the authentic path to healing requires professionals to treat the suffering mind within the context of the embodied person. It is only when the fundamental humanity of the patient is acknowledged and honored that the stigma can be dismantled, effective therapeutic alliances can be forged, and true, lasting recovery can begin.

# Conclusion

Outside, the screens of Neo-Paris flashed with the usual chaos. A new climate refugee crisis in the south, a drone strike in the east, a scathing expose on corporate tax havens, and an ever-louder chorus of identity movements, each splintered into increasingly specific, often mutually aggressive, factions. An advocate, a climate policy strategist with a decade of scars, had dedicated her life to these battles. She'd marched for equality, lobbied for economic justice, and spent countless nights wrestling with data, trying to prove, beyond a shadow of a doubt, that the planet was dying, and we were killing it.

But nothing stuck. The solutions, clear as day on paper, faltered in execution. People weren't just disagreeing; they weren't listening. They were reacting, projecting, lashing out from a place of profound internal disquiet. Facts bounced off walls of pre-existing beliefs, nurtured by algorithmically perfected echo chambers. Empathy was a weakness, nuance a luxury.

It's not the policies. It's the minds that are meant to enact them, or defy them. We're trying to build a cathedral on quicksand.

We see it everywhere: the climate deniers, not just ignorant, but clinging to a narrative that protected them from overwhelming grief; the economic disparity, not solely about greed, but about a frantic, almost pathological drive for security born of deep-seated scarcity fears; the identity wars, not just about rights, but about validation, belonging, and the fierce, often desperate need to be seen in a world that feels increasingly isolating. Even the unbearable imbalance of power, often stemmed from profoundly insecure individuals wielding authority as a shield against their own inner demons.

The problem isn't a lack of data, nor even a lack of good intentions in many quarters. It is a profound, species-wide deficit in critical thinking, fueled by a mental health crisis that boiled beneath the surface of every global issue. People weren't thinking; they were feeling, reacting, and then rationalizing, often with devastating consequences. They were ill-equipped to sit with discomfort, to challenge their own biases, to genuinely listen to a perspective that didn't immediately align with their tribe's doctrine. They were too anxious, too angry, too depressed, too triggered to approach complex issues with the clarity and collective spirit required.

The shift will begin subtly. We will stop framing arguments as "right vs. wrong" and start asking "why do we believe this?" We will organize community dialogues not around specific policy proposals, but around shared values, fears, and hopes. We will push for media literacy programs that taught not what to believe, but how to evaluate information, how to identify logical fallacies and emotional manipulation. We will advocate, not for more laws, but for more space—space for quiet reflection, for genuine debate, for accessible mental health resources that allow people to process their trauma and anxiety, rather than project it onto the nearest scapegoat.

Start small. In your local district, launch a pilot program. It isn't about recycling targets or carbon offsets, but about cultivating critical thinking. Workshops on cognitive biases, active listening exercises, facilitated discussions where participants are challenged to articulate the perspective of someone they vehemently disagreed with, not to convert, but to understand. Then pair it with accessible stress-reduction techniques and community-led mental health support groups.

The initial results will be slow, almost imperceptible. But then, something will shift. A local dispute over a new housing development, which would typically devolve into shouting matches and online vitriol, instead will see residents engage in a structured negotiation. They will still disagree, but with a newfound capacity for nuance, a willingness to compromise, and a genuine effort to understand the underlying concerns of the 'other side'. The solution they will forge isn't perfect, but it will be their solution, collaboratively built, not forced by a policy from above.

This is a colossal, generational task. The world's problems haven't vanished; the climate still warms, inequality still festers, power still consolidates. But the lens through which they were viewed will have shifted. The noise was still there, but now, a fragile, hopeful counter-melody will emerge: the quiet hum of minds, finally learning to think. Not just about the external threats, but about the internal landscape that shaped their response to everything. Because, in my unapologetic opinion, the greatest policy any species could ever enact is the policy of understanding its own mind. The rest will follow.

The shift will not be televised, nor mandated from above. It will begin in quiet rooms, in difficult conversations, in the sacred discomfort of listening. And when it arrives, it will not feel like victory—it will feel like recognition.

# FURTHER READING

**Books on Manteno State Hospital**

• Kleen, Michael. Mysterious Manteno State Hospital. Kindle ed. N.p.: Amazon Digital Services, 2011.

• Taylor, Troy. Weird Illinois. New York: Sterling Publishing Co., Inc., 2005.

— Includes a chapter on Manteno's haunted legacy and institutional rupture.

**Selected Works by Thomas Szasz**

• Szasz, Thomas. The Myth of Mental Illness: Foundations of a Theory of Personal Conduct. New York: Harper & Row, 1961.

• ———. The Manufacture of Madness: A Comparative Study of the Inquisition and the Mental Health Movement. New York: Harper & Row, 1970.

• ———. Ceremonial Chemistry: The Ritual Persecution of Drugs, Addicts, and Pushers. Garden City, NY: Anchor Press/Doubleday, 1974.

• ———. Insanity: The Idea and Its Consequences. New York: John Wiley & Sons, 1987.

• ———. Pharmacracy: Medicine and Politics in America. Westport, CT: Praeger, 2001.

• ———. Psychiatry: The Science of Lies. Syracuse, NY: Syracuse University Press, 2008.

**Szaszian Ensemble: Authors of Sovereign Dissent**

• Foucault, Michel. Madness and Civilization: A History of Insanity in the Age of Reason.

— Ritualizes the genealogy of madness, reframing psychiatric power as historical choreography.

• Laing, R.D. The Divided Self: An Existential Study in Sanity and Madness.

— Dignifies the inner experience of psychosis, mythologizing schizophrenia as existential rupture.

• Illich, Ivan. Medical Nemesis: The Expropriation of Health.

— Critiques institutional medicine as ceremonial overreach, choreographing health as sovereign autonomy.

• Breggin, Peter. Toxic Psychiatry.

— Critiques pharmacological governance, ritualizing editorial mercy and patient sovereignty.

• Moncrieff, Joanna. The Myth of the Chemical Cure.

— Interrogates the biochemical veil, choreographing psychiatric medication as mythic metaphor.

• Gøtzsche, Peter C. Deadly Medicines and Organized Crime.

— Indicts Big Pharma with sovereign clarity, reframing medical harm as institutional choreography.

## BOOKS BY BRIAN PADJEN

Green Acre: A Novella

A Habit to Break: A Novella

Silent Waters

Le Café Bleu

A Refusal to Mourn: A Love Story

Endless Night

Flesh and Machine: The Prosthetic Wars

Hummingbirds

Whispering Pines

Oh...Mary...

My Spinning Place

Innocence and Becoming

The Great and Amazing Frank Dillard

Divestment

Where the Land Listens

Piccolo Bob

The Squircle Chronicles

[]

# Don't miss out!

Visit the website below and you can sign up to receive emails whenever Brian P Padjen publishes a new book. There's no charge and no obligation.

https://books2read.com/r/B-A-NULVD-EVAEH

BOOKS 2 READ

Connecting independent readers to independent writers.

# Also by Brian P Padjen

Hummingbirds
Oh... Mary...
Silent Waters
The Endless Night
A Refusal To Mourn
Le Cafe' Bleu
Green Acre
Flesh and Machine
Whispering Pines
My Spinning Place
The Great and Amazing Frank Dillard
Innocence and Becoming
A Habit to Break
Divestment
Where the Land Listens
Piccolo Bob
The Squircle Chronicles: Brief Testimonies From the Edge
Manteno Never Was The Problem

# About the Author

Brian Padjen is a freelance writer and poet who has published ten books in the past three years, writing across various genres to explore the existential challenges of human existence. His poetry, inspired by historical events and personal observations, has appeared in small press journals over the years. Beyond writing, Brian leads an informal book club, fostering thoughtful discussions and a shared love of literature. With master's degrees in English Literature and Clinical Psychology, he combines psychological insight with literary artistry, captivating readers and sparking introspection.

www.ingramcontent.com/pod-product-compliance
Lightning Source LLC
LaVergne TN
LVHW101613210926
848480LV00008B/354
* 9 7 9 8 2 3 2 7 4 3 4 7 5 *